MEDICAL FINALS
Passing the Clinical

Third Edition

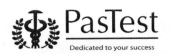

PasTest
Dedicated to your success

MEDICAL FINALS
Passing the Clinical

Third Edition

Matthew R. Todd BSc (Hons), MBBS, MRCP(UK)
Specialist Registrar in Renal & General (Internal) Medicine
Wessex Renal & Transplant Service
Queen Alexandra Hospital
Portsmouth

Christopher E.G. Moore BSc (Hons), MBBS, PhD, FRCP
Consultant Clinical Neurophysiologist
Queen Alexandra Hospital,
Portsmouth
Honorary Lecturer
University of Portsmouth

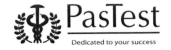

PasTest
Dedicated to your success

© 2010 PASTEST LTD
Egerton Court
Parkgate Estate
Knutsford
Cheshire
WA16 8DX

Telephone: 01565 752000

First Edition 1996
Second Edition 2005
Reprinted 2009
Third Edition 2010
Reprinted 2012

ISBN: 1 905635 70 2
           978 1905635 70 2
A catalogue record for this book is available from the British Library.

The information contained within this book was obtained by the author from reliable sources. However, while every effort has been made to ensure its accuracy, no responsibility for loss, damage or injury occasioned to any person acting or refraining from action as a result of information contained herein can be accepted by the publishers or author.

PasTest Revision Books, Intensive Courses and Online Revision
PasTest has been established in the field of undergraduate and postgraduate medical education since 1972, providing revision books, intensive study courses and online revision for doctors preparing for their professional examinations.

Books and courses are available for:
Medical undergraduates, MRCGP, MRCP Parts 1 and 2, MRCPCH Parts 1 and 2, MRCS, MRCOG Parts 1 and 2, DRCOG, DCH, FRCA, Dentistry.

For further details contact:
PasTest, Freepost, Knutsford, Cheshire WA16 7BR
Tel: 01565 752000   **Fax: 01565 650264**
www.pastest.co.uk   **enquiries@pastest.co.uk**

Text prepared by Carnegie Book Production, Lancaster

Printed and bound by CPI Group (UK) Ltd, Croydon, CR0 4YY

CONTENTS

INTRODUCTION TO THE THIRD EDITION

Medicine is constantly changing. Although we seldom see entirely new diseases the epidemiology, classification, investigation, diagnosis and treatment move forwards on an almost daily basis. Medical education, the medical curriculum and examinations are also being continually revised and updated. Our aim in the complete revision of this book for the third edition has been to keep pace with all these changes, while retaining the core concept of the book as a revision aid not a textbook. In particular, we have updated and added to the case mix and viva questions to account for the increased use of cases with mock patients/ actors, enabling many more conditions to be seen in finals.

Generally speaking the 'old' long case, short case and viva have been replaced by hopefully more objective measures of assessment, such as the objective structured long examination record (OSLER), objective structured clinical examination (OSCE) and mini clinical evaluation exercise (Mini-CEX). Vivas are increasingly reserved for honours and borderline pass/fail students. However, while the methods of medical school examination have changed, the clinical examination, signs and symptoms have not. A student's ability to demonstrate competence still relies on good communication skills with the patient and examiner, an understanding of a structured clinical examination and the ability to recognise clinical signs and put them into context.

Where possible, up-to-date guidelines from National Institute for Health and Clinical Excellence (NICE) and the learned societies have been followed or précised – however, medicine is an art as well as a science, and there are few hard-and-fast rules that can be applied in all circumstances. Guidelines are not laws, and consideration of the patient in front of you should always be foremost in your mind. In many cases local practice is guided by local issues, such as the prevalence of antibiotic resistance in various populations.

Each case in this book gives the main clinical features that may be present and some of the associated findings. The longer cases include features you may glean from the history. We have concentrated on cases which are common or important in clinical practice, favourites for exams, or archetypes for a range of less common diseases. We have labelled some of the more obscure cases as hard (rare/advanced/honours) so that valuable time is not wasted starting with these.

The '**Comments**' give some associated and hopefully relevant facts. Many of these may be needed to answer extra questions during the clinical or in any viva voce.

As always, we hope you find the book useful and wish you luck in the examination and your future careers.

THE PATIENTS

INPATIENTS

Most patients will have stable conditions and will not be very unwell at the time of the examination. You will not see someone on the day they experience a myocardial infarction but you may see them a few days later before discharge, especially if they have a murmur, rub or evidence of heart failure. While 'on the wards' try to get a feel for the kind of patients who would be suitable/well enough for transfer to another ward on the morning of the examination.

OUTPATIENTS

In the weeks before examinations the consultants and their medical teams are asked to look for patients with noteworthy physical signs in our clinics and to ask them if they would come in to help with examinations. This is often a prime time to attend extra clinics as part of your revision. Many consultants and medical schools keep lists of patients with stable clinical signs who are regularly called up to help with undergraduate and postgraduate examinations.

ACTORS

Actors are increasingly used to assess history-taking skills. The 'patient' will have been well versed in a history with positive findings for you to elicit and the clinical features of the particular disorder (eg the headache of raised intracranial pressure secondary to a space-occupying lesion), and will give you the 'right' answers if you ask for them.

The actor may have been instructed to come across as tense, irritable, tearful, etc, especially if the primary focus is on your communication skills – the 'difficult consultation'. Be prepared for this, and do not allow yourself to feel intimidated. If the actor asks you difficult questions, don't guess. Politely say that you are uncertain, but that you will ask advice from your senior colleagues. You are being examined on your competence to take up a position as a foundation year one junior doctor, not a consultant physician!

MODELS

Certain clinical skills (eg passing a nasogastric tube), intimate or uncomfortable examinations (eg digital rectal examination, fundoscopy) may be performed on models or simulators rather than volunteers. There may or may not be an actor present as well for you to interact with (eg obtaining verbal consent), but in either case you must remember to treat the model as if it were a real patient, explaining the procedure as you go, giving any instructions required, thanking them at the end and protecting their dignity. Don't worry about looking silly, and don't miss out on easy marks by forgetting to introduce yourself to a plastic arm!

STATIONS WITHOUT PATIENTS

Some medical schools include radiography, electrocardiography, prescribing, etc in their clinical finals examinations. As with clinical stations, the key is to have a well-rehearsed systematic approach.

In all cases, practise on the wards, with your colleagues and doctors, and remember the words of Sir William Osler: 'He who studies medicine without books sails an uncharted sea, but he who studies medicine without patients does not go to sea at all.'

HOW TO USE THIS BOOK AND PASS

Buy your own copy! This allows us to increase our retirement fund and you to scribble all over it.

Use the syllabus checker to find the gaps in your knowledge and confidence.

Revise with others. Get one of your colleagues to choose a case (without telling you what it is) and go through the relevant history-taking/ systems examination(s) having them tell you what you would find. Learn to synthesise the findings as you go, eg a patient presenting with breathlessness with clubbing should have you thinking of fibrotic lung disease/bronchiectasis/bronchial carcinoma before you reach for the stethoscope.

Practise, practise, practise. It is obvious to both patients and examiners when a candidate is not familiar with a certain aspect of the examination. Get used to being observed by practising in front of your peers, as well as junior and senior doctors.

Seek out patients with relevant conditions and review their signs.

Think of a patient with long-standing diabetes and a full house of complications: how many cases can you cover?

Find out as much as you can about your medical school's exam structure from previous (successful) candidates. Are you allowed to talk during the cases? Can you describe your findings as they arise or must you wait to the end and then present the full picture?

Learn how to be a confident (not arrogant) human being. This will facilitate your interpersonal skills and therefore your technique in the examination.

ACKNOWLEDGEMENTS

FIRST EDITION

We would like to thank the many colleagues who have given useful tips while producing this book and especially those who have taught us over the years, in particular:

Stephen Brecker, Senior Registrar, Cardiology; Terry Wardle, Consultant Physician; Jon Shaffer, Senior Lecturer, Gastroenterology; George Lipscombe, Senior Registrar, Medicine; Andy Higham, MRC Training Fellow; Matthew Lewis, Registrar, Gastroenterology; Wolfgang Schady, Senior Lecturer, Neurology; Tony Heagerty, Professor of Medicine; Claire Pulford, Lecturer, Geriatric Medicine; Chris Rickards, Senior Registrar, Neurology; David Neary, Professor of Neurology; Eve Russell, Senior Registrar, Psychiatry; Peter Goulding, Consultant Neurologist; Mike Davies, Senior Lecturer in Medicine; Malcolm Littley, Consultant Physician; Mohammed Akil, Senior Registrar, Rheumatology.

Responsibility for the accuracy of this text is of course our own. We would also like to acknowledge the support of our families:

Teddy, Dan, Lucie, Matthew and Keith.

SECOND EDITION

Many people have helped us over the past 7 years in the progression of our careers both as clinicians and as researchers and personally. Of our colleagues not previously mentioned Dr David McKee, consultant neurologist, wrote the HIV case for us. We thank Drs Mark Roberts, Ruth Seabrook, Claire Pulford, Angelica Wiek, David Holder, Peter Heath, Max Lyons-Nandra and Louis Merton. Kath, Julie, Anna, Jo, Gill, Christina, Pauline, Julie and Trudy also deserve mention.

We are pleased with the continued support of PasTest, in particular Lorna Young, Nicky Paris and Kirsten Baxter whose patience has been much appreciated. We would also like to acknowledge the support of friends and family, in no particular order: Keith, Matthew, Joe, Dan, Teddy, Cheryl, Charlotte, James, Lila, Gill, Sarah, Richard, Thomas, Will, Alex, Ben and Matty.

I would like to dedicate my efforts to the memory of my father Michael who sadly died a few years ago (CM).

THIRD EDITION

I would like to thank all the doctors who have taught and inspired me throughout my undergraduate and specialist training, especially but not exclusively Janet Porter, David Oliveira, Colin Borland and Menna Clatworthy. I am indebted to my parents and family for their continued support and encouragement. Many medical students and doctors have helped with ensuring that the coverage in this book is representative of medical finals examinations across the country, including Angela Etheridge, Ben Irving and Ryan Buchanan. Special thanks to my study buddies who got me through my own finals with copious tea and cake-of-the-day – Jordan Durrant and Mark Salmon. (MT)

I would again like to thank my family and friends for their support and the Portsmouth Hospital Review Team without whom I would not have met the talented Dr Todd. (CM)

We also thank Cathy Dickens at Pastest for help and advice, Dr Lanny Cucumber for his usual inspiration and all at Costa Coffee (PHT). Thanks to Philippa Fabb for writing the case on Obstructive Sleep Apnoea and Tim Cassford for the Headache case. Both also helped enormously with proof-reading, suggestions and alterations.

ABBREVIATIONS

Common abbreviations are listed below. Other abbreviations are explained where they first appear.

ABG	arterial blood gas
ACE	angiotensin-converting enzyme
ACTH	adrenocorticotrophic hormone
ADH	antidiuretic hormone
ADLs	activities of daily living
AF	atrial fibrillation
AIDS	acquired immune deficiency syndrome
AKI	acute kidney injury
ALT	alanine transaminase
AMA	anti-mitochondrial antibody
AMTS	Abbreviated Mental Test Score
ANA	anti-nuclear antibody
ANCA	anti-neutrophil cytoplasmic antibody
APTT	activated partial thromboplastin time
ARB	angiotensin receptor blocker
AS	aortic stenosis
AST	aspartate transaminase
AV	atrioventricular/arterio-venous
BiPAP	biphasic positive airways pressure
BMI	body mass index
BP	blood pressure
BTS	British Thoracic Society
CABG	coronary artery bypass graft
CCF	congestive cardiac failure
CKD	chronic kidney disease
CLO	campylobacter-like organism (*H. pylori*)
CMV	cytomegalovirus
CNS	central nervous system
COCP	combined oral contraceptive pill
COPD	chronic obstructive pulmonary disease
CPAP	continuous positive airways pressure
CRP	C-reactive protein

CT	computed tomography
CVA	cerebrovascular accident (stroke)
CVS	cardiovascular system
CXR	chest radiograph
DC	direct current
DCM	dilated cardiomyopathy
DKA	diabetic ketoacidosis
DNA	deoxyribonucleic acid
dsDNA	double-stranded DNA
DVLA	Driver and Vehicle Licensing Agency
DVT	deep vein thrombosis
EBV	Epstein-Barr virus
ECG	electrocardiogram
eGFR	estimated glomerular filtration rate
ENT	ear, nose and throat
ESR	erythrocyte sedimentation rate
FBC	full blood count
FEV$_1$	forced expiratory volume in 1 second
FSGS	forcal segmental glomerulosclerosis
FSH	follicle stimulating hormone
FVC	forced vital capacity
GH	growth hormone
GI	gastrointestinal
GORD	gastro-oesophageal reflux disease
GTN	glyceryl trinitrate
GU	genito-urinary
HGV	heavy goods vehicle
HHT	hereditary haemorrhagic telangiectasia
HIV	human immunodeficiency virus
HOCM	hypertrophic obstructive cardiomyopathy
HONK	hyperosmotic non-ketotic coma
HRCT	high-resolution CT scan (of the chest)
HRT	hormone replacement therapy
HTN	hypertension
IBD	inflammatory bowel disease
ICU	intensive care unit
IGF-1	insulin-like growth factor 1
IHD	ischaemic heart disease
ILD	interstitial lung disease

INR	international normalised ratio
iv	intravenous
IVC	inferior vena cava
JVP	jugular venous pressure
LA	left atrium
LBBB	left bundle branch block
LDH	lactate dehydrogenase
LFT	liver function test
LH	luteinising hormone
LIF	left iliac fossa
LKM	liver-kidney microsomal antibody
LLQ	left lower quadrant
LLSE	lower left sternal edge
LMWH	low molecular weight heparin
LTOT	long-term oxygen therapy (at home)
LUQ	left upper quadrant
LV	left ventricle
LVF	left ventricular failure
LVH	left ventricular hypertrophy
MC&S	microscopy, culture, sensitivity
MCV	mean cell volume
MI	myocardial infarction
MR	mitral regurgitation
MRI	magnetic resonance imaging
MS	multiple sclerosis
MSE	mental state examination
MSk	musculoskeletal
NHS	National Health Service
NICE	National Institute for Health and Clinical Excellence
NSAID	non-steroidal anti-inflammatory drug
OGD	oesophago-gastro-duodenoscopy
OSA	obstructive sleep apnoea
PCI	percutaneous coronary intervention
PE	pulmonary embolism
PEFR	peak expiratory flow rate
PET	positron emission tomography
PND	paroxysmal nocturnal dyspnoea
PPI	proton pump inhibitor
PSC	primary sclerosing cholangitis

PT	prothrombin time
PTH	parathyroid hormone
PVD	peripheral vascular disease
QOL	quality of life
RA	rheumatoid arthritis
RBBB	right bundle branch block
RDW	red cell distribution width
RhF	rheumatoid factor
RIF	right iliac fossa
RLQ	right lower quadrant
RUQ	right upper quadrant
RV	right ventricle
RVF	right ventricular failure
RVH	right ventricular hypertrophy
SBP	spontaneous bacterial peritonitis
sc	subcutaneous
SIADH	syndrome of inappropriate antidiuretic hormone
SLE	systemic lupus erythematosus
SMA	smooth muscle actin antibody
SOB	shortness of breath
SSRI	selective serotonin reuptake inhibitor
SVC	superior vena cava
SVCO	superior vena caval obstruction
TB	tuberculosis
TCA	tricyclic antidepressant
TED	thromboembolic deterrent
TFT	thyroid function test
TIA	transient ischaemic attack
TIPSS	transjugular intrahepatic porto-systemic shunt
TSH	thyroid stimulating hormone
TVF	tactile vocal fremitus
U&E	urea and electrolytes
US	ultrasound scan
VDRL	Venereal Disease Research Laboratory (test for syphilis)
VSD	ventricular septal defect
VTE	venous thromboembolism
WBC	white blood cell (count)

SYLLABUS CHECKER

As an aid to revision you can use this syllabus as your own personal checklist. You should aim to achieve at least two ticks per case before the date of the examination. * = Hard cases.

		Confidence		
		Low	Medium	High
Communication skills				
	History taking	☐	☐	☐
	Assessing cognition	☐	☐	☐
	Difficult consultations	☐	☐	☐
	Smoking cessation	☐	☐	☐
Cardiovascular system				
	Examination	☐	☐	☐
1	Acute coronary syndrome	☐	☐	☐
2	Hypertension	☐	☐	☐
3	Heart failure	☐	☐	☐
4*	Pericarditis/pericardial effusion	☐	☐	☐
5	Venous thromboembolic disease	☐	☐	☐
6	Infective endocarditis	☐	☐	☐
7	Atrial fibrillation	☐	☐	☐
8	Mitral stenosis	☐	☐	☐
9	Mitral regurgitation	☐	☐	☐
10	Aortic stenosis	☐	☐	☐
11	Aortic regurgitation	☐	☐	☐
12	Mixed mitral valve disease	☐	☐	☐
13	Mixed aortic valve disease	☐	☐	☐
14	Tricuspid regurgitation	☐	☐	☐
15	Prosthetic heart valves	☐	☐	☐
16*	Complex congenital heart disease	☐	☐	☐
17	Ventricular septal defect	☐	☐	☐
18	Measuring the blood pressure	☐	☐	☐
19	ECG interpretation	☐	☐	☐
20*	Pacemakers	☐	☐	☐
21	Resuscitation station	☐	☐	☐

		Confidence		
		Low	Medium	High
Respiratory system				
	Examination	☐	☐	☐
22	Obstructive lung disease	☐	☐	☐
23	Interstitial lung disease	☐	☐	☐
24	Pneumonia	☐	☐	☐
25	Bronchial carcinoma	☐	☐	☐
26	Cystic fibrosis	☐	☐	☐
27	Pleural effusion	☐	☐	☐
28	Superior vena caval obstruction	☐	☐	☐
29	Old tuberculosis	☐	☐	☐
30*	Sarcoidosis	☐	☐	☐
31	Pneumothorax	☐	☐	☐
32	Obstructive sleep apnoea	☐	☐	☐
33	Presenting a chest radiograph	☐	☐	☐
34	Inhaler technique	☐	☐	☐
35	Arterial blood gas interpretation	☐	☐	☐
Abdominal system				
	Examination	☐	☐	☐
36	Chronic liver disease	☐	☐	☐
37	Inflammatory bowel disease	☐	☐	☐
38	Altered bowel habit	☐	☐	☐
39	Upper gastrointestinal bleed	☐	☐	☐
40	Anaemia	☐	☐	☐
41	Acute kidney injury	☐	☐	☐
42	Chronic kidney disease	☐	☐	☐
43	Solid organ transplant	☐	☐	☐
44	Nephrotic syndrome	☐	☐	☐
45	Hepatomegaly	☐	☐	☐
46	Splenomegaly	☐	☐	☐
47	Hepatosplenomegaly	☐	☐	☐
48	Ascites	☐	☐	☐
49	Renal masses	☐	☐	☐
50	Digital rectal examination	☐	☐	☐

		Confidence		
		Low	*Medium*	*High*
51	Passing a nasogastric tube	☐	☐	☐
52	Urine dipstick testing	☐	☐	☐

Endocrine system

53	Diabetes mellitus	☐	☐	☐
54	Obesity and the metabolic syndrome	☐	☐	☐
55	Hyperthyroidism/Graves' disease	☐	☐	☐
56	Hypothyroidism	☐	☐	☐
57	Cushing's syndrome	☐	☐	☐
58	Addison's disease	☐	☐	☐
59	Acromegaly	☐	☐	☐
60*	Panhypopituitarism	☐	☐	☐
61*	Hyperparathyroidism	☐	☐	☐
62	Examination of thyroid status	☐	☐	☐

Musculoskeletal system

	Examination	☐	☐	☐
63	Rheumatoid arthritis	☐	☐	☐
64	Systemic lupus erythematosus	☐	☐	☐
65	Multiple myeloma	☐	☐	☐
66	Osteoarthritis	☐	☐	☐
67	Osteoporosis	☐	☐	☐
68	Systemic sclerosis	☐	☐	☐
69	Ankylosing spondylitis	☐	☐	☐
70	Paget's disease	☐	☐	☐
71	Gout	☐	☐	☐
72	Clubbing	☐	☐	☐
73	Upper limb nerve lesions	☐	☐	☐

Neck

	Examination	☐	☐	☐
74	Goitre	☐	☐	☐
75	Lymphadenopathy	☐	☐	☐
76	Jugular venous pressure	☐	☐	☐

		Confidence		
		Low	Medium	High

Skin

		Low	Medium	High
	Examination	☐	☐	☐
77	Psoriasis	☐	☐	☐
78	Eczema/dermatitis	☐	☐	☐
79	Cellulitis	☐	☐	☐
80	Neurofibromatosis	☐	☐	☐
81	Dermatomyositis/polymyositis	☐	☐	☐
82	Erythema nodosum	☐	☐	☐
83	Pyoderma gangrenosum	☐	☐	☐
84	Pre-tibial myxoedema	☐	☐	☐
85	Necrobiosis lipoidica	☐	☐	☐
86	Erythema ab igne	☐	☐	☐
87*	Erythema multiforme	☐	☐	☐
88	Vitiligo	☐	☐	☐
89	Pityriasis versicolor	☐	☐	☐
90*	Hereditary haemorrhagic telangiectasia	☐	☐	☐
91	Bullous skin disease	☐	☐	☐

Nervous system

		Low	Medium	High
	Examination of the arms	☐	☐	☐
	Examination of the legs	☐	☐	☐
	Examination of the cranial nerves	☐	☐	☐
92	Cerebrovascular accident	☐	☐	☐
93	Multiple sclerosis	☐	☐	☐
94	Epilepsy	☐	☐	☐
95	Headache	☐	☐	☐
96	Parkinson's disease	☐	☐	☐
97*	Motor neurone disease	☐	☐	☐
98*	Myotonic dystrophy	☐	☐	☐
99*	Myasthenia gravis	☐	☐	☐
100	Syringomyelia	☐	☐	☐
101	Spastic paraparesis	☐	☐	☐
102	Myopathy	☐	☐	☐
103	Peripheral neuropathy	☐	☐	☐

		Confidence		
		Low	*Medium*	*High*
104	Pes cavus	☐	☐	☐
105	Absent ankle jerks, extensor plantars	☐	☐	☐
106	Gait abnormalities	☐	☐	☐
107	Cerebellar syndrome	☐	☐	☐

Visual fields

108	Homonymous hemianopia	☐	☐	☐
109	Bitemporal hemianopia	☐	☐	☐
110*	Central scotoma	☐	☐	☐
111	Tunnel vision/concentric constriction	☐	☐	☐

Pupils

112*	Horner's syndrome	☐	☐	☐
113*	Holmes–Adie pupil	☐	☐	☐
114*	Argyll Robertson pupil	☐	☐	☐

Eye movements

115	Nystagmus	☐	☐	☐
116*	Internuclear ophthalmoplegia	☐	☐	☐
117	Nerve III lesion	☐	☐	☐
118	Ptosis	☐	☐	☐
119	Nerve VI lesion	☐	☐	☐
120	Thyroid eye disease	☐	☐	☐
121*	Strabismus	☐	☐	☐

Fundi

122	Fundoscopy	☐	☐	☐
123	Diabetic eye disease	☐	☐	☐
124	Hypertensive eye disease	☐	☐	☐
125	Optic atrophy	☐	☐	☐
126	Papilloedema	☐	☐	☐
127	Retinal pigmentation	☐	☐	☐

| | | Confidence | |
| | Low | Medium | High |

Other cranial nerves

		Low	Medium	High
128	Facial nerve (VII) palsy	☐	☐	☐
129*	Cavernous sinus syndrome	☐	☐	☐
130*	Cerebello/pontine angle lesions	☐	☐	☐
131*	Jugular foramen syndrome	☐	☐	☐
132	Bulbar palsy	☐	☐	☐
133	Pseudobulbar palsy	☐	☐	☐
134	The 3 Ds	☐	☐	☐

Psychiatry

		Low	Medium	High
	Examination	☐	☐	☐
135	Depression	☐	☐	☐
136	Assessing suicidality	☐	☐	☐
137	Psychosis/schizophrenia	☐	☐	☐
138	Eating disorders	☐	☐	☐
139	Substance abuse	☐	☐	☐

Therapeutics

		Low	Medium	High
140	Writing a drug chart	☐	☐	☐
141	Reporting an adverse event	☐	☐	☐
142	Overdose	☐	☐	☐
143	Human immunodeficiency virus	☐	☐	☐

Emergency skills

		Low	Medium	High
144	Assessment of the acutely ill patient	☐	☐	☐
145	Severe sepsis	☐	☐	☐
146	Acute pulmonary oedema	☐	☐	☐
147	Acute severe asthma	☐	☐	☐
148	Hyperkalaemia	☐	☐	☐
149	Anaphylaxis	☐	☐	☐

THE LONG CASE

INTRODUCTION TO THE LONG CASE

These include traditional long cases as well as the increasingly used objective structured long examination record (OSLER), mini clinical evaluation exercise (MiniCEX) and case-based discussion (CBD).

In the traditional long case candidates are usually given 45–60 minutes to take a history from and examine a patient. This is followed by 15 minutes for presentation and discussion. Do not be surprised if you are taken back to the patient to demonstrate the physical signs you have elicited.

The OSLER, MiniCEX and CBD will have the examiner(s) present. You will be graded according to your communication skills, systematic approach and logical progression through history, examination, differential diagnosis and plan for investigations and management as well as whether you elicit the 'correct' history and signs. Although the examiner will have seen you interact with the patient you may still be expected to present an ordered and concise summary of your findings, including important positive and negative features, and you should practise this aspect thoroughly.

Your clinical note-keeping may also be examined. Ensure you allow yourself at least 5 minutes at the end of the patient's examination to prepare yourself and your notes. Write a summary of the salient features of the history and examination, and your differential diagnosis. Think about what questions regarding investigation and management you may be asked – if possible, include a management plan in your notes.

It is important to establish a good rapport with the patient. Introduce yourself, explain what you are about to do and how much time you have. Try to make the patient feel that they are on your side against the examiner – this way they will try to help you as much as possible early on. If the patient is an inpatient, find out when they were admitted and why. Often the patient will have a chronic condition: in these cases the history of presenting complaint may go back over many years and it is best to go over the history chronologically and then concentrate on the major current problems. Don't forget to ask the patient if they know their diagnosis!

You may be expected to perform a full physical examination, possibly including measurement of blood pressure and urinalysis. Occasionally the patient will have no abnormal physical signs.

If you are asked to present the case fully be clear and concise, avoiding long lists of negative findings. Volunteer a short summary at the end rather than wait to be asked. Be prepared, however, for the examiner to plough straight in instead with questions regarding your differential diagnosis and management plan. A good start may be one such as this: 'I have been to see Mrs Smith, a 53-year-old lady who is currently an inpatient at this hospital under the care of Professor Jones.' Then either: 'She was well until two weeks ago when she presented with acute central chest pain...' or 'She has a 15-year history of rheumatoid arthritis and was admitted last week for investigation of anaemia...'

Some cases may be pure history-taking and discussion. Others may be a full, focused systems examination with minimal opportunity for talking to the patient. Find out the various formats in your finals examinations/ attachment assessments. Above all, be prepared!

Be courteous at all times – to patients and examiners alike.

LONG CASE INDEX

Listed below are popular long cases that appear frequently in examinations. Those in **bold** have histories covered in detail in this book as they are the most common/important.

THE SHORT CASE

INTRODUCTION TO THE SHORT CASE

These include traditional short cases as well as the increasingly used objective structured clinical examination (OSCE).

In traditional short cases you may be taken round a variable number of cases by (usually) two examiners. The cases will last a few minutes each, but are not necessarily of a fixed length – once the examiners are happy that they have assessed your competence in the relevant area, they will move on to the next case. The types of case will usually be balanced between the systems – it would be unusual for a candidate not to be asked to examine the cardiovascular system, for example.

OSCEs are relatively rigid in their structure, timing and mark scheme. Each candidate in a particular OSCE 'circuit' will see the same cases as the others, and usually each examiner stays at one station for the entire exam. This has the advantage that, even if one station goes particularly badly, the following stations are being assessed by examiners who did not witness the bad performance!

You will be assessed on:

> Your approach to the patient
> Your ability to perform a structured, competent examination
> Your ability to pick up important signs
> Your ability to interpret these signs

Your approach to the examiners is not formally tested but, if good, can only help in their overall assessment of you.

There will be marks available for your consideration of the patient. It is VERY important that you are polite, introduce yourself, wash/disinfect you hands (eg alcohol gel) and obtain verbal consent before you examine them, respect their dignity and do not hurt them. Do not lose these easy marks.

APPROACH TO THE PATIENT

A good start may sound like this:

> Examiner: 'Please examine this man's heart.'

> Candidate (making good eye contact with the patient and shaking their hand): 'How do you do, sir? I am Mr Smith. Would it be alright if I examined your heart?'

> Patient: 'Yes.'

> Candidate: 'Please would you take off your top and lean back against the pillows. Are you comfortable? I'm just going to take a step back and have a good look to start with...'.

APPROACH TO THE EXAMINERS

On first meeting the examiners make sure you introduce yourself. Try to answer the question asked and not something else. You may be encouraged to keep a running commentary, or to examine silently and then present. You may be allowed to continue uninterrupted or be stopped and started – this can be frustrating, but if you are prepared for it you should not allow it to disrupt your routine. Practise examining and presenting in all these ways throughout your revision – the only thing you want to be doing for the first time on the day of the exam is passing!

When you have finished examining the patient, thank them, make sure they are covered and comfortable and then turn to face the examiners. Good eye contact and posture help to present a competent appearance. Look at the spot at the top of the examiner's nose and let rip! 'On examining Mr Smith's cardiovascular system I found evidence of mitral regurgitation without mitral stenosis which is not complicated by infective endocarditis or heart failure, as evidenced by...'.

If you are unsure of the diagnosis try: 'I am uncertain about the definitive diagnosis but my differential diagnosis is that of an ejection systolic murmur. Aortic stenosis is unlikely as the pulse character is normal, mitral regurgitation may be present but there is no radiation to the axilla. The other possibility is aortic sclerosis, which is common in a man of this age.'

THE SPOT DIAGNOSIS

Don't be surprised if, instead of being asked to go through the examination of a system, you are simply asked to look at a patient, or perhaps ask them some questions and then come up with the diagnosis. Don't panic.

Certain conditions lend themselves to spot diagnosis, and tend to come up again and again. Often these are either endocrine or neurological conditions. Most should be familiar to you; if not, make sure you recognise them from picture atlases or find patients with them on the wards or in clinics.

Classic spot diagnoses:

55 Graves' disease

56 Hypothyroidism

57 Cushing's syndrome

58 Addison's disease

59 Acromegaly

68 Systemic sclerosis

69 Ankylosing spondylitis

70 Paget's disease

80 Neurofibromatosis

90 Hereditary haemorrhagic telangiectasia

96 Parkinson's disease

98 Myotonic dystrophy (dystrophica myotonica)

99 Myasthenia gravis

THE VIVA

The viva can be a very frightening experience as the whole of the medical syllabus is up for discussion. This is usually made worse by your supposed friends, who often do their best to 'psych' you out in the days and minutes leading up to the event.

A few tips are listed below that can make things easier during the examination. There are several ways of gaining valuable experience during your clinical training:

Arrange to have a mock viva

Act as a helper if your hospital runs an MRCP course or PACES examination

Ask the consultants teaching you about their favourite viva questions

Ask previous candidates about their experiences (common topics as well as the rarities and horror stories!)

During the viva:

Use good body language (eye contact/posture)

Speak clearly/do not mumble

Answer the question asked

If you do not understand the question, say so at once

If you know nothing about the subject under discussion, say so at once – you will either be given a clue or the subject will be changed

Don't be afraid to take a breath and pause before answering

If in doubt about something, return to first principles (if you can remember them)

Make sure you know the management of emergency situations (see case 144)

When asked for the management of Condition X always start with the ABCs then return to the well-worn path of history – examination – bedside investigations – simple blood tests – specific blood tests – simple radiology/investigations – specific radiology/investigations – conservative treatment (including patient education) – medical treatment – surgical treatment – palliative/symptomatic treatment. For example:

Examiner: 'How would you manage a patient with pneumonia?'

Candidate: 'I would ensure that the patient was safe by checking the airway, breathing and circulation and resuscitating as appropriate. As long as they were stable, I would confirm the diagnosis by taking a full history and examination, checking the vital signs and temperature, and taking blood for an FBC, U&Es, LFTs and inflammatory markers. If there was suspicion of an atypical pathogen I would request specific serology. I would request a chest radiograph looking for evidence of consolidation. Treatment would be directed at supporting the patient with oxygen and eradicating the infection with antibiotics...'

You should follow this schema every time a similar question is asked – soon the examiner will pre-empt you by saying something like 'You've already checked the ABCs and confirmed your diagnosis with history and examination...'. At this point you have already won half the battle.

When asked for causes of a particular condition, go through your medical sieve (VITAMIN D):

V Vascular

I Infective (bacterial/viral/fungal/other)

T Traumatic

A Autoimmune/connective tissue

M Metabolic/endocrine

I Iatrogenic/idiopathic

N Neoplastic (benign/malignant/primary/secondary)
Neuropsychiatric

D Degenerative/ageing

When asked to describe a particular condition, use the following:

Dressed	Definition (one sentence if possible)
In	Incidence/prevalence
A	Age
Surgeon's	Sex
Gown	Geography
Anaesthetists	Aetiology
Perform	Pathology (macroscopic/microscopic)
Deep	Diagnostics (history/examination/ investigations (simple to complex))
Coma	Clinical features/complications
To	Treatment (conservative/medical/ surgical/palliative)
Perfection	Prognosis

When asked about complications, think through each body system in turn (use the same schema as for review of symptoms (ROS) in History Taking – p. 4):

CVS	Heart, blood pressure, peripheral vessels
Resp	Lungs, upper airways
GI	Upper GI, lower GI, hepatobiliary, nutritional
GU	Renal, urinary, gonadal, anogenital
Neurology	Brain, cranial nerves, peripheral nerves, eyes, ears
MSk	Skin, joints, muscles
MSE	Mood, behaviour, cognition, social functioning
Other	Haematological, immune

When in doubt, take a breath, collect your thoughts and try to break the question down into manageable chunks. Classify and subclassify, ie 'The management of X can be broken down into investigations and treatment. Investigations may be for diagnosis, classification, or to rule out complications. Diagnostic investigations include...'. This buys thinking time and ensures a structured answer in which you are unlikely to miss anything.

As in any examination a degree of good luck always helps. We hope your quota arrives on the day – good luck.

The cases

COMMUNICATION SKILLS

Communication skills: history-taking

Presenting complaint (PC)
History of presenting complaint (HPC)
Past medical history (PMH)
Family history (FH)
Social history (SH)
Drug history (DH)
Review of systems (ROS)
Summary

PC   Remember to use the patient's words – not your interpretation of them. Patients rarely complain of melaena/haemoptysis/dysarthria, etc.

HPC   Try to start with open questions: 'Tell me about your cough.'

Focus the questions: 'When did you first notice it?'; 'Has it been getting better or worse?'; 'What is your sputum like?'

Ask for specifics with closed questions: 'Is there any blood?'

For each symptom you need to ascertain, where relevant:

Site of pain/paraesthesia, etc.

Onset   Sudden or gradual; duration

Character of pain/let patients use their own words

Radiation   'Does the pain go anywhere else?'

Associated symptoms, eg pain, breathlessness, nausea

Timing   When do the symptoms occur? Continuous/variable/episodic? Frequency of episodes?

Exacerbating/relieving factors

Severity, eg 1–10 scale or 'What does it stop you doing?'

Once you have questioned the patient fully regarding the PC, specifically ask the other questions relating to that particular organ system, eg if patient complains of shortness of breath, ask specifically about cough, sputum (colour, consistency, amount, haemoptysis), fever, chest pain

PMH   Ask about past medical/surgical/psychiatric histories
HTN/diabetes/asthma/tuberculosis/rheumatic fever

FH 'Is there anything that runs in the family?'

Record details of all first-degree relatives (parents/siblings/children)

Record the age at death/cause of death/related illnesses

SH Smoking: current/ex-smoker/never smoked

How much, how many years – pack-years?

Alcohol: regular/occasional/binge drinker/abstinent

Approximate units per week

Occupation and previous occupations/unemployment

Income support/Invalidity benefit/Other allowances

Home situation: 'Who else is at home with you?'

Relationships: married/single/divorced/widowed

House/bungalow/flat/steps, and driving ability

Activities of daily living – washing, dressing, eating, shopping; do any home help/carers/family help?

DH Use generic names rather than brand/proprietary names

Dose/dose frequency/duration of prescribed medication

Record recent changes in medication, especially those made during this inpatient stay

Ask specifically about allergies and their nature

Ask about over-the-counter/herbal/alternative remedies

ROS Briefly ask questions pertaining to each organ system:

CVS: chest pain, orthopnoea, PND, palpitations

Respiratory: breathlessness, wheeze, cough, sputum

GI: bowel habit, appetite, weight loss, nausea/vomiting

GU: difficulty passing urine, pain/stinging, continence

Neurological: weakness, numbness, fits, faints, blackouts, eyes, ears

Musculoskeletal: aches, pains, stiffness in the muscle, joints or back

MSE: how are you in yourself?

Ask about the patient's concerns with regard to their symptoms and try to find out if they have any specific worries relating to potential diagnoses or the impact illness may have on their life

Summary: Try to summarise the important positive findings rather than repeat the whole history.

Communication skills: assessing cognition

This may be necessary if a patient (or relative) complains of memory difficulties, or if during the history you get a contradictory or muddled account. A brief assessment of short- and long-term memory is the Abbreviated Mental Test Score (AMTS). If time allows, and you have a pen and paper, the more comprehensive Mini-Mental State Exam (MMSE) can be used.

If a patient can't clearly answer your questions consider also if there is dysphasia (expressive/receptive) or dysarthria (case 134).

AMTS

Tell the patient you are going to ask some questions to check his or her memory. Explain that some of the questions may seem basic.

Orientation in time, place and person:

What **day** of the week is it today?	1
What is the **month**?	1
What **year** is it?	1
What is the name of this **building** we're in?	1
What is your **date of birth**?	1
What's my **job?** And this person?	1

Long-term memory:

What was the year that **World War II** started?	1
Who is the current **Prime Minister**?	1

Recall and concentration:

Give the patient an address to remember (42 West Street) and ask him or her to repeat it back to you so you know that he or she has heard correctly.

Start at **20** and count down to one	1
What was that **address** I told you?	1

Record the score out of 10, and comment on which area of memory is affected by any deficit.

Both the AMTS and the MMSE are *screening* tools not *diagnostic* tools.

They do not distinguish dementia, acute confusion or appropriate disorientation such as after a prolonged period of sedation on the intensive care unit. Take the patient's culture, language and physical situation into account.

MMSE

Orientation in time (5 points)
> Year, month, day of the week, date, time of day

Orientation in place (5 points)
> Country, county, town, building, floor

Registration (3 points)
> Name three objects and ask the patient to repeat them (orange, plane, tiger)

Concentration (5 points)
> Ask the patient to Spell 'WORLD' backwards or to subtract 'Serial 7s' (100 − 7, − 7, …)
> (D-L-R-O-W or 100, 93, 86, 79, 72, 65)

Recall (3 points)
> Ask the patient to repeat the objects named previously

Language (2 points)
> 'What is this called?' (Point to a watch) 'And this?' (A pen)

Reading and writing (2 points)
> (Write the phrase 'Close your eyes' on a piece of paper)
> Ask the patient to 'Do what it says on the piece of paper'
> 'Please write down a sentence – it can be anything you like'

Repetition (1 point)
> Ask the patient to repeat the phrase: 'No ifs, and/or buts.'

Three-stage command (3 points)
> 'Take this piece of paper in your left hand (1), fold it in half (1), and give it back to me (1)'

Complex processing (1 point)

   (Draw two interlocking pentagons) 'Copy this picture'

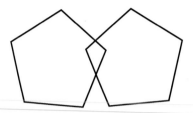

A score of >26/30 is normal; remember to adjust the score if the patient is unable to perform part of the test, eg visual impairment.

Communication skills: difficult consultations

This covers a wide range of possible situations: breaking bad news, dealing with a complaint or angry patient/relative, and explaining and apologising for a medical or other error.

Preparation

   Hand your bleep over to someone else

   Find a suitable private area where you won't be disturbed

   Have a third party present (eg nurse involved with the patient's care)

Introduction

   Explain who you and your colleague(s) are

   Find out to whom you are talking – relationship to patient

   Ask them if they would like someone else present

Background

Ask what is already known about the situation

Elicit their concerns, fears or dissatisfactions

Let them talk – listen non-judgementally, try not to interrupt or explain at this stage; acknowledge any anger

Explanation

Apologise if there has been an error or omission

Try to state the diagnosis/problem clearly and non-technically

Questions

Encourage questions and clarify any unclear points

Check understanding, eg by asking the patient to summarise what you have said

Follow-up

What will you need to do now?

Is there any further information that the patient would like?

If you cannot provide it now, clarify how and when you will, eg further investigation

What does the patient need to do now?

Does the patient need to discuss anything with family?

Further appointment/formal complaints procedure

Documentation

Say that you would clearly document the consultation including who was present and the outcome

Communication skills: smoking cessation

Brief interventions by healthcare professionals improve the chances of patients achieving lifestyle changes. The basic format of a brief intervention for smoking cessation can be applied to other areas, such as reducing alcohol intake and dietary or exercise advice.

Assess the current situation

Do you smoke? How much do you smoke?

Assess willingness to change

> Have you thought about stopping smoking? Would you like to try stopping?
>
> If the patient does not want to stop, encourage him or her to think about it, and briefly state the benefits. Don't labour the point!

Highlight benefits in a change of behaviour

> Concentrate on the positive aspects of stopping, rather than the negative aspects of continuing
>
> Health benefits – fitness and well-being, lifespan
>
> Financial benefits

Explain some tools that the patient can use himself or herself

> Discuss with family and friends – they may want to quit too
>
> Throw away lighters, ashtrays

Explain what support is available

> Self-help, eg with websites, leaflets, nicotine replacement
>
> NHS Free Smoking Helpline
>
> NHS Stop Smoking Services include individual counselling and stop smoking groups – what would the patient prefer?

Consider pharmacological therapy if support is declined/fails

Explain that every time they try they are more likely to succeed

The only people who can't stop smoking are those who never try

Previous 'failed' attempts are positive, not negative

Plan to review the situation in the future

VIVA QUESTIONS

What are the 'four pillars of medical ethics'?
The four principles that underpin medical ethics are:

1. **Autonomy**, respecting a patient's right to make decisions about life and care

2. **Beneficence**, acting with the intention of benefiting others

3. **Non-malevolence**, avoiding harm to the patient/others

4. **Justice**, being fair to the wider community, such as in the equitable distribution of scarce resources

How would you assess a patient's capacity to consent to a procedure?
All patients aged 16 or over are presumed to have capacity to consent unless there is evidence to the contrary. Capacity is not 'fixed' – it may vary, eg with mental state, use of intoxicants or intercurrent illness. In assessing whether a patient has capacity consider the following:

Are they able to understand the treatment/procedure that they are consenting to, and why it is being suggested?
Are they able to understand the risks–benefits involved?
Are they informed about alternatives, including not having the procedure, and what this might lead to?
Are they able to weigh this information in their mind and come to a conclusion?
Are they able to communicate their decision?

Ways of assessing this may involve explaining the procedure, alternatives and the risk–benefit of each course of action, then asking the patient to explain back to you in his or her own words.

How would you take and record consent?
Consent should be taken before any interaction with a patient, even a simple physical examination – without consent this is an assault. After ensuring that the patient had capacity, explain what you want to do and why, and ask for consent. This discussion could be recorded on a consent form, although this is merely a record of the process of achieving consent and does not mean that consent has been irretrievably given. A patient can withdraw consent at any time.

CARDIOVASCULAR SYSTEM

Examination of the cardiovascular system

Introduce and expose
Patient comfortable, reclining at 45°

Observe Pallor
Dyspnoea/cyanosis

Hands	Clubbing (case 72)	Cyanotic heart disease
	Splinter haemorrhages	Endocarditis
	Peripheral cyanosis	Cool peripheries
	Tendon xanthomas	Hyperlipidaemia
	Tar staining	Vascular disease
	Smoking	

Pulse Rate and rhythm at the radius
Radiofemoral delay in young adults (case 2)
Check for collapsing pulse (case 11)

Blood pressure (case 18)
Tell the examiner 'I would like to measure the blood pressure'. If you are lucky you will be told what it is

Neck Carotid pulse for character
JVP (case 76)
↑ + pulsatile in RVF (case 3)
↑ + non-pulsatile in SVCO (case 28)
Waveform
Giant systolic V waves in tricuspid regurgitation (case 14)
May displace ear lobes

Face Pallor (anaemia)
Xanthelasma
Corneal arcus
Malar flush

With patient sitting back,

Praecordium

Inspect	Scars	Median sternotomy
		CABG/valve replacement
		Lateral thoracotomy (mitral valvotomy)
		Apex visible
	Palpate	Localise apex beat
	Tapping	Palpable valve closure
	Heaving	Sustained contraction
	Thrusting	Hyperdynamic contraction
	Thrills	systolic murmurs – AS (case 10), MR (case 9)
		Parasternal heave – RV hypertrophy
Percuss	Not usually performed	
Auscultate		

Time any murmurs with the carotid pulse

1. At apex with bell
2. Turn patient on to left-hand side

    Relocate apex and listen specifically for mitral stenosis (case 8) in held expiration

    Turn patient back
3. At apex with diaphragm

    If murmur listen for radiation into axilla
4. Listen in all other areas:

    Lower left sternal edge (tricuspid)

    Upper left sternal edge (pulmonary)

    Upper right sternal edge (aortic)
5. Listen to carotids (If no aortic murmur, ? isolated carotid bruit)

With patient sitting forward,

Praecordium
> Listen specifically for the early diastolic murmur of aortic regurgitation (case 11) at the lower left sternal edge in held expiration

Lungs Listen at lung bases for inspiratory crackles

Sacrum Feel for sacral oedema while asking the patient 'Does this hurt?' This should alert the examiner to the fact you have looked for sacral oedema

Feel for ankle oedema and note any vein harvest sites (CABG)

Tell the examiner
> 'To finish my examination I would like to see the temperature chart and dip the urine' (? endocarditis)

When presenting your findings comment on the valve lesion(s) and whether it is complicated by heart failure (case 3) or endocarditis (case 6), eg 'This woman has mitral stenosis, as evidenced by the mid-diastolic murmur heard loudest at the apex in held expiration, which is complicated by atrial fibrillation but not heart failure or endocarditis'.

COMMENT

Left-sided murmurs increase in held expiration, right-sided with inspiration.

ACUTE CORONARY SYNDROME

Remember that stable angina is not an acute coronary syndrome. Unstable features (new chest pain, increasing frequency or severity of attacks, or brought on by less than the usual exertion or at rest) can be unstable angina (without a cardiac enzyme rise), non-ST-elevation myocardial infarction (NSTEMI), or ST-elevation MI (STEMI).

PC	**Chest pain** (usually; can be just neck/arm/jaw or none)
	Sometimes no chest pain but SOB/collapse/sweating
HPC	Pain **Central**/radiation to neck/jaw/teeth/arms (one or both, usually LEFT)
	Crushing/squeezing/tight/'like a band'
	May be described with a clenched fist at the sternum (Levine's sign)
	Occasionally felt as radiation only
	Typically at rest/may be brought on by unusual exercise/argument/intercourse/snow shovelling, etc.
	Pain is prolonged/often relieved only by opiate analgesia
	Poorly relieved by GTN
	Associated symptoms include SOB/sweating/nausea/vomiting/pallor/greyness/impending doom
	Ask about any chest pain or SOB since admission
PMH	Ask about previous vascular disease:
	Stable angina – present in about 40%
	Claudication
	Cerebrovascular disease
	Hypertension/high cholesterol/diabetes
FH	Particularly a history of ischaemic heart disease in a first-degree relative

SH   **Smoking habit** – before admission

Employment may be profoundly affected, eg large goods vehicle or passenger carrying vehicle drivers are banned from driving if follow-up exercise test reveals abnormal findings after full-thickness infarct

DH   Before and since admission

Was the patient put on a drip (thrombolysis)?

Did he or she have an angiogram/stent (primary PCI)?

Is he or she now on aspirin/clopidogrel/both?

ROS   Chest pain/SOB, orthopnoea, PND/ankle swelling

EXAMINATION

General appearance

Anaemia/xanthomas/xanthelasma/corneal arcus/tar staining/pyrexia

CVS   Atrial fibrillation (case 7) (common post-MI)

Bradycardia (heart block/β-blocker treatment)

Blood pressure often low post-MI

Presence of fourth heart sound very common

Look for signs of left ventricular failure:

Poor cardiac output/basal crackles/dyspnoea

Evidence of peripheral vascular disease:

Absent pulses/femoral bruits/carotid bruits

INVESTIGATIONS

An ECG should be taken as soon as possible on presentation

Troponin I/T levels ('cardiac enzymes')

FBC

CRP/ESR

(Both WBC count and inflammatory markers may be elevated)

U&Es/glucose

Cholesterol (within 24 hours of MI)

Chest radiograph

ECG FINDINGS (MAY BE NORMAL)

Acute full-thickness infarct (STEMI):

>ST elevation >1 mm in limb or >2 mm in chest leads
>(Anterior V1–4; lateral V5–6, I, aVL; inferior II, III, aVF)
>New left bundle branch block (LBBB)

NSTEMI/acute angina:

>ST depression, T-wave inversion, lesser ST changes

TREATMENT

Immediate treatment with MONA:

M	Morphine/opiate analgesia
O	Oxygen to maintain SaO_2 94–98% (88–92% in COPD)
N	Nitrates (sublingual/iv)
A	Anticoagulation (aspirin, clopidogrel, LMWH)

Definitive treatment with PCI/thrombolysis for STEMI

Stop smoking

SEQUELAE

Early   Cardiac arrhythmias
Heart failure (case 3)
Pericarditis (case 4)
Recurrent infarction/Post-infarct angina
Left ventricular thrombus
Mitral regurgitation (chordae rupture) (case 9)
Ventricular septal/free wall rupture

Late   Heart failure (case 3)
Dressler's syndrome (4)
Ventricular aneurysm

COMMENT

Advice to give patient on discharge after an MI:

Stop smoking

Dietary changes (less meat, fat and salt, more fish, fruit and vegetables)

Weight reduction if overweight/obese

Exercise sufficient to increase exercise tolerance, eg a cardiac rehabilitation programme. Aim for 20–30 min/day

Sexual intercourse once able to walk without discomfort

Avoid driving for 4 weeks (you need not inform the DVLA)

Avoid flying for 2 weeks or until symptoms are controlled

Most patients should aim to return to work within 2–3 months

Some occupations that may be affected:

large goods vehicle/passenger carrying vehicle/public service vehicle driving

Airline pilot

Unless contraindicated, all patients should be on aspirin, a statin, a β-blocker and an ACE inhibitor

The patient may present with complications of HTN or be asymptomatic. Examination focuses on identifying any underlying cause, other metabolic and CVS risk factors, and any end-organ damage.

PC   Often none

If malignant HTN: headaches, vomiting, cardiac failure, AKI

Symptoms of cardiovascular disease: angina, SOB

HPC   How long has the patient been known to be hypertensive?

Paroxysms of flushing, tachycardia, palpitations (phaeochromocytoma)

PMH   Cardiovascular, cerebrovascular, peripheral vascular disease

Diabetes

FH   Commonly present

SH   Smoking

Heavy alcohol use

Liquorice, salt intake

Psychological stress

Physical activity

DH   Antihypertensives, including diuretics

Primary/secondary prophylaxis for IHD, eg aspirin, statins

Drugs causing HTN: NSAIDs, oral contraceptives, steroids

ROS   Angina, claudication

SOB, orthopnoea, PND

Ankle swelling

Muscle weakness, polyuria (Conn's syndrome)

EXAMINATION

General appearance

In a younger patient look for underlying causes of HTN

Endocrine causes: Cushing's disease, acromegaly, thyroid disease

Habitus

CVS Pulses in both wrists (radioradial delay: coarctation proximal to the left subclavian)

Blood pressure in both arms

Signs of LVH: forceful, sustained non-displaced apex (pressure overload)

Respiratory

Signs of LVF: pulmonary oedema

Abdominal

Ballot the kidneys

Check for an abdominal aortic aneurysm

Listen for renal bruits (renovascular disease)

Peripheries

Check for radiofemoral delay on both sides

Femoral bruits (peripheral vascular disease)

INVESTIGATIONS

Examine the fundi: papilloedema/retinal haemorrhage may indicate malignant HTN

ECG, echocardiogram looking for LVH

Urine dipstick: haematuria/proteinuria suggesting primary renal disease

U&Es   Low K^+ in Conn's syndrome; chronic kidney disease as cause/consequence

Blood sugar, cholesterol

Serum renin:aldosterone ratio (Conn's syndrome)

Urinary catecholamines (phaeochromocytoma)

TREATMENT

Lifestyle changes; treat any underlying cause
Antihypertensive drugs: A(B)/CD approach
Consider aspirin, statins for primary CVS prevention

SEQUELAE

Vascular disease: IHD, CVA, PVD
Hypertensive heart disease: LVH, heart failure
Hypertensive nephropathy
Hypertensive retinopathy
Hypertensive encephalopathy

HEART FAILURE

Heart failure can be classified by which side of the heart it affects (LVF/RVF), the phase of the cardiac cycle (systolic/diastolic), the haemodynamics (low output/high output) or whether the main problem is failure to clear pre-load or failure to generate a perfusing pressure (backward/forward failure).

PC Breathlessness (due to: pulmonary oedema, LVF; effusions, RVF; unable to raise cardiac output on demand)
Ankle swelling (RVF, CCF)

HPC SOB better on sitting upright/at rest
Exercise tolerance
Orthopnoea (how many pillows does the patient sleep on?)
PND
Cough, sputum – white/pink, frothy/watery
Change in weight (fluid retention), girth (ascites)

PMH IHD, previous MI (case 1)
Hypertension (case 2)
Chronic lung disease (cor pulmonale, RVF)
Cardiomyopathy (see below)

SH Heavy alcohol use (DCM)
Smoking

DH Previous chemotherapy (DCM)
ACE inhibitors, ARBs, β-blockers
Diuretics, eg furosemide, spironolactone, thiazides

ROS Chest pain, claudication

EXAMINATION

Introduce and expose

Observe	Dyspnoea/oedema	
	Hands	Cool/peripheral cyanosis
	Pulse	Tachycardia/poor volume
	BP	Low
	Neck	JVP raised (case 76), may be behind ear

Praecordium

	Palpate	Displaced apex beat (volume overload)
	Auscultate	Third ± fourth heart sounds
		Functional murmurs of mitral and/or tricuspid regurgitation
	Lung bases	Inspiratory crackles/pleural effusion
	Abdomen	Pulsatile smooth hepatomegaly
	Sacral oedema	
	Ankle oedema	Yes – may extend as far as trunk/chest wall

INVESTIGATIONS

ECG If completely normal, heart failure is unlikely
Evidence of old IHD
Atrial/ventricular hypertrophy or conduction defects

Chest radiograph

Cardiomegaly, pulmonary oedema, pleural effusions
Echocardiogram to assess ventricular systolic (and diastolic) function and regional wall motion abnormalities (ie old MI), and to exclude valve disease and septal defects
Consider investigation for other causes of SOB, eg PEFR

TREATMENT

For acute pulmonary oedema see case 146

Diuretics

Vasodilators, eg intravenous GTN, for acute LVF

ACE inhibitors, spironolactone, β-blockers (once stable)

COMMENT

Causes:

LVF	IHD
	Cardiomyopathy (dilated/restrictive/HOCM)
	Volume overload (eg mitral/aortic regurgitation)
	Pressure overload (eg aortic stenosis, HTN)
RVF	Most commonly LVF (back-pressure)
	IHD (right ventricular MI)
	Volume overload (eg septal defect)
	Pressure overload (eg pulmonary HTN/stenosis)

Arrhythmias can both cause and complicate heart failure, eg AF reduces ventricular filling by the atria, and can be caused by a stretched, volume-overloaded atrium.

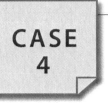

CASE 4

PERICARDITIS AND PERICARDIAL EFFUSION

The patient may have pain, signs of heart failure, or both. You should know the signs of tamponade, although this is unlikely to be present in a patient well enough to be used in an exam.

PC	Pleuritic pain, classically relieved by sitting forward
	Symptoms of heart failure (see case 3)
	Fever (infective/autoimmune including Dressler's syndrome)
	Acute trauma, including rib fractures
HPC	Timing of symptoms – onset, duration
	Recent viral illness
	Recent MI, cardiac intervention/surgery
	Recent chest infection (parapneumonic/empyematous)
PMH	Chronic kidney disease (uraemic pericarditis)
	Systemic autoimmune disease, eg lupus (polyserositis)
DH	Anticoagulation – risk of pericardial haemorrhage
ROS	· SOB, orthopnoea, PND
	Ankle swelling

EXAMINATION

General appearance

JVP may be elevated; rise in JVP with inspiration in tamponade

CVS	Blood pressure may be low (especially with tamponade)
	Recent sternotomy scar (Dressler's syndrome)
	Quiet heart sounds and indistinct apex beat (see case 16)
	Pericardial rub (not necessarily present with large effusions)

Respiratory

> Signs of LVF: pulmonary oedema
>
> Pleural effusion(s):
>
> > Unilateral – ? infection/malignancy causing pericarditis
> >
> > Bilateral – ? polyserositis/transudates, eg CCF, nephrosis

Peripheries

> Peripheral oedema
>
> Ask to see the temperature chart (viral pericarditis) and the urine dipstick (nephrosis)

INVESTIGATIONS

ECG Small complexes with large effusions

'Saddle-shaped' ST elevation diffusely → globally, reciprocal depression aVr/V1

PR-segment depression, especially laterally, reciprocal elevation in aVr

Electrical alternans with a large effusion

Chest radiograph

> Enlarged, globular heart with loss of left atrial window

FBC May have raised WBC

CRP Raised if inflammatory, normal suggests CCF/nephrosis/myxoedema

LFTs Albumin low in inflammatory states/nephrosis

Cardiac enzymes

> May be modestly elevated, exclude MI

Echocardiogram is the investigation of choice

TREATMENT

> Treat underlying mechanism of effusion, eg NSAIDs (inflammation), diuretics (CCF)
>
> Pericardiocentesis to relieve tamponade/for diagnosis

SEQUELAE

Constrictive pericarditis (causing restrictive cardiomyopathy)

COMMENT

Dressler's syndrome is a pericarditis putatively caused by an autoimmune reaction to pericardial/myocardial antigens released after damage from an MI or cardiac surgery. It can occur days or weeks after the injury and usually resolves spontaneously with supportive treatment and anti-inflammatories.

VENOUS THROMBOEMBOLIC DISEASE

DVT and PE are common conditions, and can be the primary illness leading to hospital admission or, more commonly, arise as a complication during hospital admission, eg post-MI, surgery.

PC Calf pain/swelling (DVT)
Breathlessness/pleuritic chest pain (PE)

HPC Gradual progression over a few days (DVT)
Sudden-onset respiratory symptoms (PE)
Ask about preceding risk factors, eg immobility, fracture
Is the patient pregnant?
Ask specifically about haemoptysis

PMH Previous DVT/PE?
History of a 'white leg' in pregnancy?

FH Very important; certain clotting deficiencies are familial

SH Smoking (see Comment)

ROS Is the patient taking COCP/HRT?
Since admission, has patient been on daily subcutaneous injections (LMWH/heparin), or tablets given at tea-time (warfarin)?

E X A M I N A T I O N

General appearance

Bruising (iatrogenic) especially at injection sites (abdomen)
High BMI

Legs Calf asymmetry (measure at the tibial tuberosity)
Tenderness over the deep veins
Erythema
Oedema, especially above the knee

CVS Sinus tachycardia (often the only sign of a PE)
High JVP with giant V waves if massive/chronic PEs
(see case 76)

Respiratory
Tachypnoeic
Oxygen treatment
Pleural rub

INVESTIGATIONS

Coagulation screen (PT/APTT) before treatment
If recurrent, seemingly unprovoked or positive family history
perform detailed thrombophilia screen
Doppler ultrasonography of calf
D-dimer if low clinical suspicion (to **rule out** not rule in)
If PE suspected need spiral CT pulmonary angiogram (CTPA) or
ventilation–perfusion ($\dot{V}/\dot{Q}$) scan
ABG: often hypoxia/hypocapnia but can be unhelpful

ECG FINDINGS (MAY BE NORMAL)

Sinus tachycardia – most common abnormality
Right ventricular strain: RBBB, right axis, $S_I Q_{III} T_{III}$ pattern

TREATMENT

Anticoagulation, initially with subcutaneous LMWH until
warfarin is therapeutic (INR >2.0), for at least 3 months (may be
lifelong if recurrent VTE)
In PE subcutaneous treatment should continue for a minimum
of 5 days, and until warfarin has been therapeutic for >24 h

COMMENT

All hospitalised patients should have their risk of VTE assessed, balanced against bleeding risk and given appropriate prophylaxis. Medical patients likely to have reduced mobility for 3+ days and most surgical patients should have pharmacological prophylaxis (LMWH/heparin). If bleeding risk is high, foot pumps/pneumatic compression/TED stockings can be used instead, or caval filters if the risk of VTE is high.

Some studies have found smoking to be an independent risk factor for VTE, and others have not – in contrast with arterial thrombosis (eg MI), where it is clearly a risk. However, it is relevant because a reduced respiratory reserve in smokers may contribute to morbidity with PEs.

CASE 6

INFECTIVE ENDOCARDITIS

An uncommon condition, but patients are usually in hospital for several weeks, and therefore appear relatively frequently in exams.

PC   Fever, constitutional symptoms

Symptoms of cardiac failure (case 3)/embolisation

HPC   Characteristically in subacute infective endocarditis the symptoms are of such gradual onset that the patient often finds it impossible to date the onset of the illness

Ask about recent dental and surgical procedures, but be aware that there is no clear association with endocarditis

Fever/sweats/chills/rigors

Non-specific constitutional symptoms are often predominant:

Malaise/weight loss/anorexia/aching joints

Occasionally the condition may present with complications secondary to embolisation, eg stroke/gut infarction

PMH   Around 50% are known to have pre-existing valve disease

History of valve surgery/replacement

VSD (case 17)

Hypertrophic cardiomyopathy

Ask for history of rheumatic fever/St Vitus' dance (chorea)

EXAMINATION

General appearance

Fever/pallor/evidence of weight loss

Petechiae – trunk/limbs/mucous membranes

Splinter haemorrhages/nail-fold infarcts

Osler's nodes (pain**ful** red **pap**ules on the **pulps**)

Janeway lesions (pain**less** red **mac**ules on the **palms**)

State of teeth/? dentures

CVS   Tachycardia/heart failure

Murmur – most commonly aortic regurgitation or mitral regurgitation

Abdominal

Splenomegaly

Urinalysis

Microscopic haematuria and proteinuria

Say that you would like to examine the fundi for Roth's spots (pale-centred retinal haemorrhages)

INVESTIGATIONS

Blood cultures × 6

Common organisms include *Streptococcus viridans* or *bovis*, HACEK bacteria (see Comments), staphylococci and enterococci

Echocardiography to look for vegetations/valve damage

Transthoracic echo (TTE) may be non-diagnostic

If clinical suspicion, transoesophageal echo (TOE)

FBC   Mild normochromic/normocytic anaemia (case 40)

CRP/ESR   Elevated

ECG findings (may be normal)

May be conduction abnormalities, eg AV block, bundle-branch block, abnormal atrial/ventricular focus/ectopics

TREATMENT

Intravenous bactericidal antibiotics, eg penicillins, according to results of blood cultures

Surgery for extensive valvular damage and heart failure/ prosthetic valve infection/failure to clear infection

COMPLICATIONS

Embolisation (from the vegetations):

Stroke (case 92)

Renal infarction

Splenic infarction (splenic rub)

Roth's spots (retina)

Janeway lesions

Immune complex formation:

Osler's nodes

Glomerulonephritis (haematuria, proteinuria)

COMMENT

The organism responsible can give a clue to the cause:

α-Haemolytic *Strep. viridans*/HACEK (*Haemophilus, Aggregatibacter, Cardiobacterium, Eikenella, Kingella* spp.) from oral mucosa – poor dentition, dental procedures

Strep. bovis – gut translocation in GI mucosal lesions

Enterococci – urinary infection, catheterisation

Staphylococcus aureus – cannulation, surgical procedures, intravenous drug use

Endocarditis on prosthetic valves (case 15) accounts for up to a third of all cases. Early infection – within 2 months of surgery – carries a particularly high mortality. Established infection will cause alteration of the prosthetic valve sounds – 'muffling' them.

Intravenous drug users are at risk of developing **right-sided** endocarditis; usually the tricuspid valve is affected (case 14). Typically the patient is young, with no known history of heart disease and a fairly short history. In these cases embolisation commonly causes pulmonary infarction ± abscess formation.

Antibiotic prophylaxis is no longer routinely recommended. Current NICE guidance advises not to offer prophylaxis to those undergoing dental, upper and lower GI, ENT and respiratory, or urogenital, procedures. However, in patients at risk of endocarditis, on antibiotics and undergoing a procedure at a site of suspected infection, antibiotics likely to cover organisms that could cause endocarditis should be used.

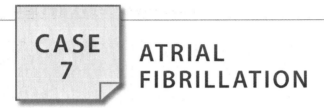

CASE 7

ATRIAL FIBRILLATION

Although atrial fibrillation (AF) may be isolated ('lone AF') be careful of associated mitral stenosis or hyperthyroidism.

Introduce and expose

Observe ? Obviously hyperthyroid

Hands	Sweating/tremor (hyperthyroidism)
Pulse	**Irregularly irregular** in rhythm and volume Ideally, count the rate over a full minute
BP	Difficult to accurately assess in AF
Neck	Goitre (hyperthyroidism) Carotid pulse JVP with absent A waves (difficult sign!)
Face	Malar flush (mitral stenosis)

Praecordium

Inspect

Palpate

Auscultate   Count the ventricular rate (compare the radial rate)

Note the varying intensity of first heart sound

Lung bases

Ankle oedema

COMMENT

Causes

1. Ischaemic heart disease
2. Mitral valve disease
3. Hyperthyroidism
4. Pneumonia/sepsis
5. Cardiomyopathy
6. Constrictive pericarditis
7. Lone AF
8. Many others

The presence of a radial–apical pulse deficit means that the AF is **uncontrolled**.

AF may be **paroxysmal, persistent** or **permanent**. In paroxysmal AF aim for **rhythm** control, eg with a β-blocker/electrical cardioversion; in the others, digoxin or a β-blocker for **rate** control.

Consider full anticoagulation with warfarin to reduce stroke risk.

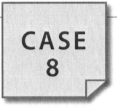

CASE 8

MITRAL STENOSIS

Introduce and expose

Observe ? Female (much more common in women)

Hands

Pulse AF (very common)

BP Low with normal pulse pressure

Neck JVP may be increased
Giant V waves of TR (case 14)

Face Malar flush (cyanosis and telangiectasia)

Praecordium

Inspect ? Left thoracotomy scar (mitral valvotomy)

Palpate Undisplaced tapping apex beat
Parasternal heave (RV hypertrophy)

Auscultate
Loud first heart sound
Opening snap
With bell, low-pitched rumbling **mid-diastolic murmur** at
apex, louder in held expiration (can be very difficult to hear)
? Pansystolic murmur at left lower sternal edge (TR)

Lung bases
Usually clear

Ankle oedema

TREATMENT

Anticoagulation to prevent systemic embolisation from LA thrombi

Diuretics for RV failure

Treat any associated AF, eg with digoxin

Mitral valvotomy/valve replacement

COMMENT

Rheumatic fever, occurring after a group A streptococcal infection, is the cause of virtually all mitral stenosis. It is thought to be an autoimmune response with antistreptococcal antibodies cross-reacting with heart, joint, skin and brain targets. It is now uncommon in the western world due to the more routine use of antibiotics for bacterial infections.

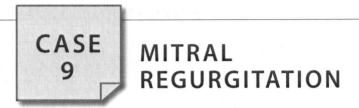

MITRAL REGURGITATION

Introduce and expose

Observe

Hands Splinters

Pulse Sinus rhythm or **atrial fibrillation**

BP

Praecordium

Inspect Visible apex beat

Palpate

    Displaced/thrusting apex beat (volume overload)

        Systolic thrill

        Parasternal heave (due to large left atrium)

Auscultate

    Soft first heart sound/third heart sound/pansystolic murmur at apex/radiation to axilla

Lung bases

    Any associated left ventricular failure?

Ankle oedema

COMMENT

Causes

1. Ischaemic heart disease
   Secondary to left ventricular dilatation (functional)
   Papillary muscle ischaemia/infarction

2. Rheumatic heart disease (previous mitral valvotomy for mitral stenosis)

3. Mitral valve prolapse

4. Infective endocarditis
   There are many others, eg the connective tissue diseases (SLE, RA), ankylosing spondylitis, Marfan's syndrome, HOCM

It is sometimes difficult to give a definitive diagnosis when listening to an ejection systolic/pansystolic murmur so be sure to work out the features of the four main differential murmurs: AS/MR/aortic sclerosis/VSD.

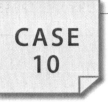

AORTIC STENOSIS

Introduce and expose

Observe Male (more common in men, see Comment)

Hands

Pulse   Sinus rhythm

BP   Low systolic with **narrow pulse pressure**

Neck   Carotid pulse   (**low volume/slow rising**/thrill)

Praecordium

Inspect   Visible apex beat

Palpate   Undisplaced **heaving** apex beat (pressure overload)
             Thrill over aortic area

Auscultate
             Harsh **ejection systolic murmur** loudest in aortic area
             Often heard easily at apex/radiates to **carotids**
             Soft second heart sound (may be absent)

Lung bases
             Normal if uncomplicated case

Ankle oedema

INVESTIGATIONS

ECG   Left ventricular hypertrophy

Echo   To assess severity (pressure gradient across valve)

Cardiac catheterisation (as a precursor to surgery)

COMMENT

Symptoms SOB/syncope/chest pain

Causes

1. Calcification of the valve (associated with atheromatous disease)

2. Bicuspid valve and degeneration

3. Rheumatic

4. Congenital (young patient)

In elderly people calcification of a normal valve can produce a murmur that is similar, but the pulse, BP and apex will be normal – so-called aortic sclerosis.

A bicuspid valve occurs in 1% of the population, and is more common in males. With increasing age the valve becomes increasingly fibrotic and calcified, and hence aortic stenosis most commonly presents in men aged 40–60 years.

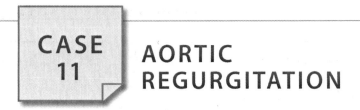

CASE 11

AORTIC REGURGITATION

Introduce and expose

Observe   Check for features of Marfan's*/ankylosing spondylitis (case 69)

Hands   Splinters/rheumatoid hands/arachnodactyly

Pulse   Sinus rhythm/**collapsing**

BP   **Wide pulse pressure**, eg 180/60 mmHg

Neck   Large volume carotid pulse/easily seen in neck

Face   High-arched palate/Argyll Robertson pupils (case 114)

Praecordium

Inspect   Visible apex beat

Palpate   Displaced/**thrusting** apex beat (volume overload)

Auscultate

         Soft/blowing **early diastolic murmur** at the left sternal edge, loudest sitting forward in held expiration

         Note that there may, in addition, be a systolic murmur due to increased flow across the aortic valve. There may also be a mid-to-late diastolic murmur (Austin Flint) due to the back flow on to the mitral valve

Lung bases

         Normal in the uncomplicated case

Ankle oedema

* High-arched palate/span > height/arachnodactyly/risk of aortic dissection/lens dislocation

COMMENT

Causes

1. Rheumatic fever
2. Infective endocarditis
3. Ankylosing spondylitis
4. Rheumatoid arthritis
5. Marfan's syndrome
6. Syphilis (aortitis)

There are a number of eponymous signs characteristic of, although rarely seen, in aortic regurgitation. They are beloved of examiners:

De Musset's sign: the head nods with each pulsation

Quincke's sign: capillary pulsation visible in the nail beds

Corrigan's sign: vigorous arterial pulsations seen in the neck

Mueller's sign: visible pulsation of the uvula

MIXED MITRAL VALVE DISEASE

It is quite common, at least in exams, to see patients with mixed mitral valve disease, ie with signs of both mitral stenosis and mitral regurgitation. Remember that, as for lone mitral stenosis, rheumatic heart disease is essentially the only cause.

Two reasons for mixed mitral valve disease:

1. Excessive valvular damage

2. Previous mitral valvotomy – **look for the lateral thoracotomy scar**

If you are doing particularly well (or you are particularly unlucky), you may be asked to comment on the predominant valve lesion:

Sign	Predominant MS	Predominant MR
Apex	Tapping	Thrusting/displaced (volume overload)
First heart sound	Loud	Soft
Third heart sound	Absent	Present
Atrial fibrillation	Common	May be present

COMMENT

Remember, the third heart sound represents rapid ventricular filling, and therefore is obviously incompatible with significant mitral stenosis.

MIXED AORTIC VALVE DISEASE

There are essentially two causes:

1. Rheumatic heart disease

2. Infective endocarditis on a previously stenotic valve

Remember, even in lone aortic regurgitation you should expect to hear a systolic murmur due to increased flow across the valve. However, there will not be any signs of aortic stenosis.

Sign	Predominant AS	Predominant AR
Pulse	Slow rising	Collapsing
Apex	Heaving (pressure overload)	Thrusting/displaced (volume overload)
Systolic BP	Low	High
Pulse pressure	Narrow	Wide

COMMENT

A bisferiens pulse is characteristic of mixed aortic valve disease.

TRICUSPID REGURGITATION

This is most commonly due to left heart failure, pulmonary hypertension or 'functional' TR from a dilated valve annulus in a volume-overloaded heart. Look for a primary cardiac (LVF, mitral stenosis, IHD) or respiratory (COPD, OSA, PEs) cause.

Introduce and expose

Observe   Track marks/Venflon sites (right-sided endocarditis)

Hands   Signs of endocarditis

Pulse

BP   May be low in congestive cardiac failure

Neck   JVP raised with giant V waves (case 76)

Praecordium

Inspect

Palpate   Parasternal heave (RV hypertrophy)

Auscultate Pansystolic murmur at left lower sternal edge

Lungs   Clear/signs of LVF/chronic lung disease

Abdomen Pulsatile hepatomegaly/ascites

Ankle oedema

COMMENT

Causes of tricuspid regurgitation

Cor pulmonale (increased pressure/resistance from lung vasculature):

  LVF, mitral stenosis

  COPD, obstructive sleep apnoea

  Chronic pulmonary infarction (chronic PEs, sickle cell disease)

  Acute pulmonary embolism (massive)

  Intra- or extracardiac shunt

  Primary pulmonary hypertension

Damaged/dilated valve apparatus:

  Congestive cardiac failure

  Dilated cardiomyopathy

  Right-sided MI

  Right-sided endocarditis, rheumatic fever

  Carcinoid syndrome

Valvular laxity:

  Rheumatoid arthritis

  Connective tissue diseases, eg Marfan's syndrome (see case 11)

  Congenital

PROSTHETIC HEART VALVES

Prosthetic valves produce a loud closing click and a quieter opening click. A flow murmur across a prosthetic valve is to be expected.

Introduce and expose

Observe Dyspnoea

Hands Splinter haemorrhages

Pulse AF (mitral valve replacement)

Collapsing pulse – aortic valve leaking

BP Wide pulse pressure – aortic valve leaking

Face Pallor (haemolysis across mechanical valve)

Praecordium

Inspect Midline thoracotomy scar (both aortic and mitral)

Palpate

Auscultate

> **Mitral valve** – loud click at first heart sound, opening click in diastole ± mid-diastolic flow murmur;
>> PSM and signs of heart failure imply valve leakage

> **Aortic valve** – normal first heart sound, ejection click, an ejection systolic flow murmur and loud click at second heart sound;
>> A collapsing pulse, wide pulse pressure and early diastolic murmur imply valve leakage

Lung bases
> Pulmonary oedema with valve leakage

Ankle oedema

COMMENT

Complications

 Endocarditis

 Emboli

 Leakage/CCF

 Mechanical dysfunction

 Haemolysis

 Bleeding due to anticoagulants

Confusion may be caused if both valves have been replaced. A valve may be replaced with a biological (human/pig) graft; this does not give rise to abnormal sounds. Always comment on whether the valve is functioning normally (a flow murmur is allowed) or whether it is complicated by leakage/CCF/endocarditis.

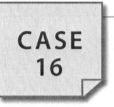

CASE 16

COMPLEX CONGENITAL HEART DISEASE

Heart defects are the most common birth defect. Most birth defects are now detected antenatally and corrected at or soon after birth. The number of defects and corrective procedures is myriad, and you will not be expected to know them all. Auscultatory findings are similarly varied, depending on the initial defect and the exact surgery performed.

Tetralogy of Fallot is the most common cyanotic congenital heart disease and is associated with 22q deletion syndromes such as DiGeorge syndrome. Total corrective surgery is now the norm.

EXAMINATION

Introduce and expose

Observe   Features of an underlying genetic syndrome

May be cyanosed if Eisenmenger's syndrome

Hands   Clubbing (case 72)

Pulse   May have poor right arm pulse if subclavian diversion (Blalock–Taussig shunt)

BP

Face

Neck

Praecordium

Inspect   May have permanent pacemaker due to arrhythmias
Midline sternotomy scar, other chest wall scars

Palpate

Auscultate
Complex and variable heart sounds and flow murmurs

COMMENT

The tetralogy is VSD, overriding aorta, pulmonary atresia and RV hypertrophy.

Infants with tetralogy often display a characteristic squatting posture because occlusion of the femoral arteries increases systemic vascular resistance and so decreases the right-to-left shunt.

The VSD component can lead to Eisenmenger's syndrome (case 17).

Corrected **transposition of the great arteries** can give a similar clinical picture.

Dextrocardia can occur in isolation or as part of situs inversus, eg with Kartagener's syndrome.

EXAMINATION

Introduce and expose

Observe Normal

Hands May be clubbed if bronchiectasis with Kartagener's syndrome

Pulse

Neck

Face

Praecordium
Inspect
Palpate Cannot palpate apex on left side
Percuss Cardiac dullness on right side
Auscultate Quiet/inaudible heart sounds (see below)

Respiratory
May have areas of bronchiectasis

Abdominal
May have liver dullness on left side

51

COMMENT

Primary ciliary dysmotility (PCD) is characterised by bronchiectasis, sinusitis and reduced fertility due to dysmotile sperm or cilia in the fallopian tubes. In PCD the cilia normally responsible for moving the shh (sonic hedgehog) gene product leftwards to create laterality are poorly motile – shh therefore moves left or right at random, with 50% having normal situs and 50% developing situs inversus, true Kartagener's syndrome.

Causes of poorly audible heart sounds/difficult apex beat:

Insulating fat	Obesity
Insulating fluid	Pleural/pericardial effusion
Insulating air	COPD/pneumothorax
Dextrocardia	Isolated/with situs inversus
Asystole	

VENTRICULAR SEPTAL DEFECT

VSD is the most common congenital heart lesion; the patient is often young. There is an association with Down's syndrome.

Introduce and expose

Observe   Young, generally well

Hands   Splinter haemorrhages (associated endocarditis)

Pulse

BP

Neck

Face

Praecordium

Inspect

Palpate   Apex undisplaced (smaller VSD)
Apex displaced (volume overload with large VSD)
Parasternal heave (RVH with large VSD)

Auscultate
Loud 'tearing' **pansystolic murmur** at left sternal edge/heard well at apex/throughout
Loud pulmonary component of second heart sound/early diastolic murmur of pulmonary regurgitation (pulmonary hypertension with large VSD)

Lung bases

Ankle oedema

COMMENT

Small VSDs (maladie de Roger) in the absence of symptoms/complications require no treatment.

Larger VSDs cause pulmonary hypertension – these cases will require cardiac catheterisation and surgical repair.

Very large VSDs can lead to Eisenmenger's syndrome, when the rising pulmonary arterial pressure causes a reversal of the shunt from left-to-right to right-to-left. The massively increased blood flow irreversibly damages the pulmonary vessels. The patient will be cyanosed with clubbing due to deoxygenated blood entering the systemic circulation. The pansystolic murmur tends to disappear as the right and left ventricular pressures equalise.

CASE 18

MEASURING THE BLOOD PRESSURE

- **Introduce** yourself and **explain** the procedure; obtain verbal consent
- Have the patient seated comfortably with the upper arm free of clothing, at heart level
- The manometer should be at eye level to avoid parallax error when recording the results
- Select an appropriately sized cuff; place snugly around the upper arm
- Palpate the radial pulse while inflating the cuff
- When the pulse is obliterated, note the BP; deflate the cuff
- Place the diaphragm of the stethoscope over the brachial artery in the antecubital fossa
- Inflate the cuff to 30 mmHg above the point where the pulse was obliterated
- Slowly deflate the cuff while auscultating over the artery
- Note the systolic BP when you first hear the pulse sounds
- Continue to slowly deflate the cuff (by about 2 mmHg per pulse beat) until the sounds completely disappear; note the diastolic BP
- Fully deflate the cuff and remove it from the patient's arm
- Record the blood pressure to the nearest 2 mmHg, along with the patient's position and which arm was used, and preferably the pulse rate (eg seated BP 138/76 mmHg, pulse 64 beats/min, left arm)
- If the patient is in AF there is no way of obtaining an accurate BP because it will vary beat to beat. Suggest that you would like to do another measurement to decrease the likelihood of a spurious result

ECG INTERPRETATION

You may or may not be provided with a brief vignette of the case. The most relevant fact is the presence or absence of chest pain.

Technical factors

Lead placement: V1 and aVR should be concordant

Amplitude: calibrated to 10 mm/mV (two large squares)

Rate: 25 mm/s (usually written at the bottom left)

Right patient, right date and time

Heart rate

R–R interval

More than six big squares: <50 beats/min, significantly bradycardic

Six big squares: 50 beats/min, bradycardic

Five big squares: 60 beats/min

Four big squares: 75 beats/min

Three big squares: 100 beats/min

Fewer than three big squares: >100 beats/min, tachycardic

Two big squares: 150 beats/min, consider atrial flutter

Causes of bradycardia: physical fitness, negative chronotropic medication (eg β-blockers), heart block, sinus node disease, Cushing's reflex

Causes of tachycardia: exercise, stress, pain, fever, sympathomimetic medication (eg salbutamol, ephedrine), hypotension, metabolic demands

Rhythm

Easiest to work out from the rhythm strip (usually lead II)

Regular, regularly irregular, or irregularly irregular

Are P waves present before every QRS complex?

Are all complexes identical or are there ectopics?

Axis

If QRS positive in leads I and aVF axis is normal

If QRS negative in lead I but positive in aVF then right axis deviation, (consider left anterior fascicular hemiblock)

If QRS positive in lead I but negative in aVF then look at lead II

If positive in lead II axis is still normal

If negative in lead II then left axis (? left posterior block)

If QRS negative in leads I and aVF then consider lead placement

P waves

Absent: AF, junctional/ventricular escape

Not always followed by QRS: ? second-degree heart block regular Mobitz type II, eg 2:1, or type II with variable block, or type I below

Large, M shaped in II, biphasic in V1: left atrial hypertrophy (mitral/aortic stenosis, hypertension)

Triangular, taller in III than I: right atrial hypertrophy (pulmonic stenosis, pulmonary HTN, cor pulmonale)

Sawtooth, rate ~300 beats/min: atrial flutter

Inverted: abnormal atrial focus

P–R interval

From start of P to start of QRS. Normal is 120–200 ms (three to five small squares):

Prolonged: first-degree AV block (with RBBB and left axis = trifascicular block – high risk of complete heart block)

Shortened: consider Wolff–Parkinson–White syndrome

PR segment depression: acute pericarditis

Lengthening P–R interval followed by dropped beat:

Wenckebach's phenomenon, Mobitz type I second-degree heart block (generally benign)

No correlation with QRS: third-degree (complete) heart block

QRS complexes

Narrow: normal; incomplete bundle branch block, ie left anterior or posterior fascicular block; if no P waves implies junctional/His bundle focus

Broad: ventricular beats/ectopics, pacemakers, high K^+

Broad, positive in V1 (may be 'M' shaped), negative in V6 (may be 'W' shaped): right bundle branch block

Broad, negative in V1 (may be 'M' shaped), negative in V6 (may be 'M' shaped): left bundle branch block (? MI)

Tall: consider left ventricular hypertrophy (S in V1 + tallest R of V5/V6 >35 mm or seven large squares)/miscalibrated

ST segments

Measured one to two small squares after the end of the QRS:

Elevated (>1 mm in limb leads, >2 mm in V1–6): acute MI (territorial), acute pericarditis (global), LV aneurysm (persistent)

Depressed: myocardial ischaemia (acute coronary syndrome, LV hypertrophy, 'rate-related' ischaemia with tachycardias), reciprocal changes with MI (If V1–V2 think posterior MI – request posterior leads)

'Sloping/slurred' depression: digoxin therapy (not necessarily toxicity), hypothermia, hypokalaemia

T waves

Normally upright except in aVR, V1, but can be inverted in V2 and occasionally V3. III may vary with respiration

Inverted: myocardial ischaemia/infarction (acute or old), ventricular hypertrophy (lateral = LV, V1–3 = RV), digoxin

Tall, 'tented', triangular: hyperkalaemia (often taller than preceding R wave)

Q–T interval

Start of QRS to end of T; needs adjusting for heart rate

As a rule of thumb, end of T should be no more than halfway between two QRS complexes – if longer than this, consider QT prolongation:

Prolonged: many drugs, congenital, hypothyroidism; risk of ventricular arrhythmias

Extra waves

> Irregular/sawtooth baseline: AF or atrial flutter
> Pacing spikes before P or QRS complexes
> U waves following T wave: hypokalaemia, thyrotoxicosis, may
> be normal

Other arrhythmias

> Ventricular fibrillation: if the patient is not arrested, this
> must be an artefact (eg tremor, tooth-brushing, electrical
> interference)
> Ventricular tachycardia
> Torsades de pointes

ECG lead territories

> Inferior: II, III, aVF
> Lateral: I, II, aVL, V5–6
> Anterior: V1–4
> Posterior: aVR, reciprocal changes in V1–3

Common diagnoses

Acute coronary syndrome (case 1)

The patient has pain. New LBBB, or territorial ST segment elevation or depression, or T-wave inversion. May be normal.

Acute pericarditis (case 4)

The patient has pain. 'Saddle-shaped' ST elevation in most to all leads. May have PR segment depression.

Left ventricular hypertrophy

High-voltage QRS complexes. May have lateral ST depression and/or T-wave inversion (without chest pain). Large P wave with 'M' shape in II and biphasic in V1. Consider HTN (case 2) and aortic stenosis (case 10).

Left ventricular aneurysm

ST elevation without pain, persisting on repeated ECGs. Risk of LV thrombus and hence embolisation and stroke, so consider anticoagulation.

Atrial fibrillation (case 7)

Irregularly irregular rhythm without visible P waves. If 'fast AF' (properly 'atrial fibrillation with rapid ventricular response') may have rate-related lateral ST depression (ask about pain).

Atrial flutter

Regular rhythm with P-wave rate of ~300 beats/min (? sawtooth appearance, though not always appreciable in every lead), QRS rate usually 150, 100, 75 or 60, ie an exact divisor of 300 (described as 2:1, 3:1, etc block). May be irregular with all R–R intervals being a whole number of large squares – 'variable block'.

Hyperkalaemia (case 148)

Long P–R interval, broad QRS, tall triangular 'tented' T waves (taller than the preceding R wave). Progresses to sine wave, then cardiac arrest. Urgent cardioprotection with calcium gluconate/chloride and then definitive treatment to reduce serum and total body potassium.

PACEMAKERS

Discussion may be sparked by a patient with a scar, a radiograph with the device visible or an ECG with pacing spikes, or when discussing arrhythmias.

Pacemaker nomenclature

Chamber paced	(V)entricle, (A)trium, or (D)ual
Chamber sensed	(V)entricle, (A)trium, or (D)ual
Sensing response	(T)riggered, (I)nhibited or (D)ual and additionally (R)ate-responsive

Single chamber pacing

VVI, VVIR – a single wire into the right ventricular apex. The pacemaker is inhibited by a ventricular impulse, ie it fires only if no autologous impulse is generated, hence it is often called a 'back-up' pacemaker. Used if no coordinated atrial activity is present, eg AF. Can be used for 'block and replace', allowing β-blockade in patients with fast AF without risk of bradycardia.

AAI, AAIR – a single atrial wire, requires intact AV–nodal and His–Purkinje conduction. Unusual, but used for sinus node disease.

Dual-chamber pacing

DDDR is the most common. Prevents the atria and ventricles contracting simultaneously, and hence the 'pacemaker syndrome'. If the atrium does not provide an impulse, the atrial lead will fire, with the ventricular lead firing only if this is not normally conducted. This allows normal, synchronous contraction of the ventricles as much as possible. Often used for heart block.

Cardiac resynchronisation therapy

Also called biventricular pacing. A wire is passed through the coronary sinus around to the outside of the left ventricle. This allows the lateral and septal (right ventricular) walls of the left heart to be activated simultaneously, leading to an improved ejection fraction in patients with dyssynchrony – wide QRS and poor (<35%) ejection fraction.

Can be CRT-P (just pacing) or CRT-D (with implantable defibrillator), as patients with dilated, dyssynchronous hearts are at risk of ventricular arrhythmias.

Implantable cardioverter–defibrillator or ICD

ICD is for patients at risk of ventricular arrhythmias but not requiring resynchronisation, eg sudden cardiac death syndromes.

Physical signs

Scar overlying pacing box, usually in left upper thorax

Pulse may be metronomically regular, eg 60 beats/min exactly (VVI)

ECG signs

None while the pacemaker is not firing:

A lead: Small pacing spikes before P waves (not necessarily visible in all leads)

V lead: Usually more prominent spikes before LBBB pattern QRS complex

Biventricular:
           QRS narrow after pacing spikes

Chest radiograph signs

- Pacing box and wires
- Atrial wire into RA, near right heart border
- Ventricular wire into RV apex, near left hemidiaphragm
- Left ventricular wire around left ventricle, near left heart border
- ICD electrodes have long areas that are thicker and more opaque than the rest of the wire

RESUSCITATION STATION

This station calls for a little theatricality – when checking the patient's responses, calling for help, etc show the examiner what you would actually do rather than simply saying 'I would call for help'. There's no harm in being loud, clear and distinct.

Is it safe to approach?

Check for responses – gently shake the patient by the shoulders while clearly asking 'Are you all right?'

Call for help – call the arrest team (eg 2222) or emergency services

Position the patient on their back (if this is safe and practical)

Open the airway (head tilt, chin lift)

Check for breathing (look, listen and feel for 10 seconds)

If you are not happy that the patient is breathing normally, declare it not normal and commence cardiopulmonary resuscitation (CPR):

- **30 chest compressions** – interlinked fingers, heel of the hand over the sternum, kneel with your shoulders over the patient and straight arms, press down 4–5 cm at a rate of 100 beats/min

- **Reopen the airway** (head tilt, chin lift); pinch the patient's nose (or cover the nose and mouth with a resuscitation mask)

- Take a normal breath and **breathe steadily into the patient's mouth**, watching to see the chest rise, for about 1 second; remove your mouth and continue head tilt, chin lift as the patient exhales

- Repeat the above for a second breath; only make two breath attempts even if one or both is ineffective

- Return **immediately** to another cycle of chest compressions

- Continue 30 compressions/2 breaths until the patient shows signs of response or help arrives

Although it is acceptable to perform compression-only CPR (100 beats/min continuous compressions), you should be able to demonstrate your ability to open and maintain an airway and administer rescue breaths.

If two people are available, one should perform compressions and one the breaths, at the same ratio of 30:2. The person performing compressions should count out loud and give clear instructions to ensure that the change between the two is as seamless as possible.

Once a defibrillator is available the cardiac rhythm should be assessed as soon as possible.

> **VT** or **VF**: give one shock (360 J or biphasic equivalent of 150–300 J depending on the defibrillator) then immediately recommence CPR for 2 min

> **Asystole** or **pulseless electrical activity**: continue CPR for 2 min; give atropine 3 mg iv as soon as possible (once only)

Recheck the rhythm every 2 min and administer shocks only if VT or VF is present.

Check for a pulse only if there is a change to a potentially perfusing rhythm, and then only during the short pause between 2-min CPR cycles – do not interrupt CPR to perform a pulse check. Give adrenaline 1 mg iv every 3–5 min, ie every other cycle.

Consider reversible causes (4 Hs, 4 Ts):

Hypoxia – give 100% O_2 via a bag–valve–mask or definitive airway (laryngeal mask/cuffed endotracheal tube)

Hypovolaemia – iv fluid to restore intravascular volume

Hyperkalaemia and other electrolyte disorders – check urgently on an ABG

Hypothermia – use a low-reading thermometer if suspected

Tension pneumothorax – if clinically present, decompress (case 31)

Tamponade – suspect if penetrating chest trauma

Toxic – if suspected, urgent bloods and definitive care directed by the toxin/drug overdose

Thromboembolism – if suspected, thrombolyse (ongoing CPR is not a contraindication)

VIVA QUESTIONS

How would you investigate and treat hypertension?

You should look for an underlying cause in any patient under the age of 20, in those under the age of 30 who require treatment, in those requiring three or more antihypertensive agents, or if the history and examination suggest a possible cause. This includes all patients with abnormal creatinine, low potassium, haematuria or proteinuria, or evidence of endocrine imbalance.

Lifestyle measures to reduce blood pressure and cardiovascular risk are indicated (stop smoking, limit alcohol, salt and fat intake, maintain a healthy weight, consume at least five portions of fresh fruit/vegetables a day, regular aerobic exercise).

If blood pressure is elevated above 160/100 mmHg, or above 140/90 mmHg with evidence of end-organ damage or high (>20% in 10 years) cardiovascular risk, drug treatment is indicated. In White patients aged under 55 years drugs affecting the renin–angiotensin–aldosterone system are preferred, ie ACE inhibitors, angiotensin receptor blockers and β-blockers. In Black patients or those aged >55 calcium-channel blockers or thiazide diuretics are first-line treatment.

What is malignant hypertension?

Malignant hypertension is extreme hypertension, often >220/120 mmHg, and causes acute vascular and end-organ damage to the eyes, brain and kidneys. It is a medical emergency and requires treatment to quickly reduce blood pressure to a safer level. Care must be taken not to drop blood pressure too dramatically because this can cause further complications such as stroke. Patients should be investigated for an underlying cause.

Give me some causes of secondary hypertension

Endocrine: Cushing's disease, Conn's syndrome, phaeochromocytoma, thyroid disease

Renal: renal artery stenosis, glomerulonephritis, CKD

Anatomical causes: coarctation of the aorta

Iatrogenic: NSAIDs, steroids, sympathomimetics

What is the NYHA classification for heart failure?

The New York Heart Association classifies by symptoms:

Class I   No limitation or symptoms with normal activity

Class II   Comfortable at rest/mild activity; little limitation

Class III Comfortable at rest, symptoms limiting activity

Class IV   Symptoms on any activity and can occur at rest

The Canadian Cardiac Society classification for angina is essentially the same, with the symptoms being chest pain rather than breathlessness.

What is the treatment of chronic heart failure?

Treatment of heart failure aims to improve symptoms and prognosis. Remember, heart failure has a worse prognosis than most cancers. It is important to exclude other contributory medical conditions, such as anaemia and thyrotoxicosis.

Lifestyle advice: regular exercise, eg cardiac rehabilitation; stop smoking; avoid alcohol if it is suspected as a cause of DCM; immunisation against pneumococci (once) and influenza (annually).

The first-line pharmacological treatment is with a diuretic, usually a loop diuretic, such as furosemide. ACE inhibitors should be used in left ventricular systolic dysfunction (care in AS), and cardioselective β-blockers added once the maximum tolerated ACE inhibitor dose is reached (care in asthma). Spironolactone can be added if symptoms persist.

Arrhythmias should be treated and warfarin given if AF is present; in permanent AF digoxin is used as it is a positive inotrope. Look for valvular disease, which might be causing the heart failure, especially AS – valve replacement is the treatment. Cardiac resynchronisation (biventricular pacing) or transplantation may rarely be necessary.

Why might you give diuretics to a patient with heart failure and a low blood pressure?

The heart's contractility increases with increased filling (Starling's law) – but only to a point; an over-filled heart will become increasingly inefficient as contractility reduces, and eventually atrioventricular valve annuli dilate, leading to 'functional' mitral/tricuspid regurgitation. Diuretics can paradoxically increase cardiac output and blood pressure by reducing volume overload.

When would you anticoagulate someone with AF?
The risks and benefits of anticoagulation with warfarin need to be assessed. AF carries a risk of systemic embolisation of thrombus formed in the left atrial appendage, commonly causing stroke. However, full anticoagulation carries a bleeding risk, particularly in those with a history of GI bleeding, falls or alcohol excess.

The need for full anticoagulation with warfarin can be assessed by using a clinical risk prediction score such as the $CHADS_2$ score, to help guide the risk-benefit of anticoagulation. The score is:

Chronic cardiac failure?   1 point if present

Hypertension?   1 point if present

Age?   1 point if >75 years old

Diabetes mellitus?   1 point if present

Stroke or TIA previously?   2 points if present

A score of 0 is low risk and should be treated with aspirin. A score of 1 is intermediate risk and the clinician and patient can make a choice between aspirin and warfarin based on preference, lifestyle factors, etc. A score of 2 or more gives a stroke risk of >4% per year, and full anticoagulation should be considered unless contraindicated.

In preparation for an attempted DC cardioversion, all patients, even those with low $CHADS_2$ scores, should be anticoagulated to an INR of >2.0 for 6 weeks before the procedure to prevent embolisation.

What can you tell me about rheumatic fever?
Acute rheumatic fever can follow an infection with a group A β-haemolytic streptococcus. It can present with a constellation of variable symptoms, thought to be due to antibody against the bacteria cross-reacting with various organ systems. The modified Duckett Jones diagnostic criteria are used: two major, or one major plus two minor criteria make the diagnosis.

Major criteria

    Migratory polyarthrits

    Peri-/myo-/endocarditis

    Erythema marginatum

    St Vitus's dance, also called Sydenham's chorea

    Subcutaneous nodules over tendons/extensor surface

Minor criteria

    Fever

    Arthralgia without arthritis

    Raised inflammatory markers

    Leukocytosis

    Heart block on ECG

    Serological evidence of recent streptococcal infection

Treatment is with anti-inflammatories (may require steroids), eradication of any infection and ongoing antibiotic prophylaxis to prevent further streptococcal infections causing relapse.

How would you grade a murmur heard on auscultation?

The prominence of a murmur can be graded from 1 to 6:

    1   Audible only with special effort in quiet surroundings

    2   Quiet, may require special effort

    3   Easily audible

    4   Loud

    5   Associated with a weak thrill (systolic murmurs only)

    6   Associated with a strong thrill (systolic murmurs only)

However, the prominence of a murmur does not necessarily correlate with the severity of the underlying lesion, eg the murmur of AS may be quiet due to low flow across a critically stenosed valve.

What is the benefit of the D-dimer test in suspected venous thrombosis/embolism?

The D-dimer test identifies cross-linked fibrin degradation products in patients with thrombosis/embolism. However, although it is sensitive (95%) it is not very specific (50%), meaning that it has a low positive predictive value. The test is most commonly used together with clinical risk scoring systems such as Wells' criteria for DVT/PE. If a patient is low risk, a negative D-dimer effectively rules out thromboembolic disease.

How would you treat deep vein thrombosis?

The main reason for treating DVT is to prevent PE.

Most commonly, LMWH is used, which has the advantage of not requiring monitoring. For patients at high risk of bleeding, however, 'standard' unfractionated heparin is more suitable, because its effects can be rapidly terminated by stopping the infusion.

Oral anticoagulation with warfarin should be started at the same time as LMWH – warfarin takes at least 48–72 hours for its anticoagulant effect to develop fully, and it is slightly procoagulant when first administered. When the INR has been in the therapeutic range (2.0–3.0) heparin can be stopped and warfarin continued, usually for a period of 3–6 months.

All patients should be given an anticoagulant card, informing them of the risks and what to look out for (spontaneous excessive bruising, bleeding) and how to seek help.

Warfarin has many drug interactions and it is important that patients are aware that they have to inform all concerned medical practitioners, dentists, etc of their prescription.

THE RESPIRATORY SYSTEM

Examination of the respiratory system

When asked to examine the chest there are only a few possible diagnoses and you should be able to differentiate between them fairly easily. However, many candidates look ill prepared when it comes to the exam. It is very important to have a strict, well-practised routine. The examination has six main parts.

Introduce and expose

Ask the patient to remove their top clothing (preserve modesty)

Patient comfortable, reclining at 45°

Observe   Dyspnoea/Respiratory rate

Ask the patient to take two deep breaths; look for:

1. Asymmetry of chest movement
2. Stridor
3. Cachexia
4. Accessory muscle use/pursed lips

Hands   Clubbing (case 72)   Chronic infection, lung fibrosis (case 22), bronchial carcinoma (case 25)

Steroidal skin   Asthma, COPD, lung fibrosis

Tar staining   Smoking

Check for asterixis (flapping tremor) – ask the patient to extend the arms and cock the wrists back (demonstrate for them)

Asterixis CO_2 retention

Fine tremor β_2 Agonists/aminophylline

Pulse   Hyperdynamic/tachycardia

Hypertrophic pulmonary osteoarthropathy (case 72): tender on squeezing wrist (usually clubbed)

Neck   Trachea pulled to side of collapse/pushed away from mass/fluid

JVP (case 76):

↑ + pulsatile in cor pulmonale (case 3)

↑ + non-pulsatile in SVCO (case 28)

Waveform: giant systolic V waves – ? pulmonary HTN

Lymphadenopathy – best felt from behind (see below)

Face

Central cyanosis – look at underside of tongue
Cushingoid
Horner's syndrome (case 112) – apical lung tumour

Chest You have to decide whether to examine the front or the back first. We would suggest the back as usually all the possible signs will be there; if so, you may be told to omit the front, thus saving valuable time and not boring the examiner.

Sit the patient forward

Inspect Scars – from lung surgery, pleural drains, phrenic nerve crush

Palpate Feel for lymphadenopathy in the cervical chains, horizontal ring and supraclavicular fossae
Expansion – make sure that your thumbs are not touching the chest

Percuss Top to bottom including axillae; compare right with left at each level
Tactile vocal fremitus (TVF) – use the ulnar border of both hands

Auscultate
Top to bottom as before
Vocal resonance (VR)

TVF and VR give the same information. Pick one and use it consistently so that you can recognise and interpret abnormal signs.

Ankle oedema

Extras Oxygen
Nebulisers/Inhalers
Sputum pot:
Pus = infection/bronchiectasis
Blood = tumour/infection
Temperature chart

COMMENT

At the end of the examination you should be in a position to make a differential diagnosis of the lung pathology. Try also to note whether there is right heart failure (cor pulmonale), eg 'This woman is breathless at rest and has signs of lower zone fibrosis consistent with a diagnosis of fibrotic lung disease. There is no evidence of right heart failure' or 'The raised JVP and ankle oedema suggest that this has been complicated by pulmonary hypertension'.

OBSTRUCTIVE LUNG DISEASE

Acute (reversible) obstructive lung disease is asthma. Chronic obstructive pulmonary disease (COPD) may be due to chronic asthma but is more commonly due to loss of lung elasticity, tissue and mucociliary clearance due to smoking and/or α_1-antitrypsin deficiency.

PC	**SOB**
	Chronic bronchitis – daily cough/sputum for at least 3 months per year for at least 2 consecutive years
	Wheeze
HPC	Breathless on effort/at rest – exercise tolerance
	Worse in circumstances:
	Time of day/time of year ('winter bronchitis')
	At work (weekdays vs weekends/holidays)
	Sputum volume, colour, consistency (? haemoptysis)
	Fever
PMH	Asthma
	Regular chest infections
	Previous hospital admissions – ever on ICU?
FH	Early lung disease (? α_1-antitrypsin)
SH	**Smoking** (number of pack-years)
DH	Any inhalers? Regular or as required? Nebulisers?
	Previous courses of oral steroids
	Oxygen at home? Long term or as required?
ROS	Weight loss, sleep disturbance

EXAMINATION

General appearance
Tar staining
Young – ? α_1-antitrypsin deficiency
Pursed-lip breathing/cyanosis/plethora
Tachypnoea, respiratory effort – accessory muscles?

Respiratory
Signs of hyperexpansion
Decreased cricosternal distance
Increased AP chest diameter (barrel chest)
Decreased expansion
Hyperresonance to percussion
Quiet heart sounds/poorly palpable apex beat
Downward displacement of the liver
Prolonged expiratory phase of breathing
Expiratory polyphonic wheeze

Extras
Signs of cor pulmonale – ankle oedema, raised JVP
Sputum pot

INVESTIGATIONS
FBC   Polycythaemia if chronic hypoxia, ? infection
Eosinophilia may be present in atopic
asthma
CRP   ? Infective exacerbation
ABG   ? CO_2 retention
Guide O_2 therapy in COPD
Tiring patient in acute asthma – beware!
Sputum for MC&S
Chest radiograph
PEFR
Spirometry – low FEV_1 with low/normal FVC = low ratio
ECG   Signs of right-heart 'strain', eg RBBB

Chest radiograph findings

May be normal

Hyperinflated – flat hemidiaphragms, long thin mediastinum

Increased lung markings

Bullous emphysema

TREATMENT

Stop smoking

Immunisations: annual flu, pneumococcus once only

Asthma

For acute severe asthma see Emergency skills, p. 359

Keep a symptom and PEFR diary to identify exacerbants

Formal spirometry and trial of treatment if diagnostic doubt

Avoid β-blockers and NSAIDs

Stepwise treatment increased/decreased as necessary:

1. Inhaled short-acting β agonists as required
2. Add regular inhaled steroid
3. Add regular long-acting β agonist
4. Consider leukotriene antagonist/theophylline
5. Oral steroids

COPD

Post-bronchodilator spirometry to confirm diagnosis

Short-acting bronchodilators as required:

Long-acting β/muscarinic agonist if FEV_1 >50%

Add inhaled corticosteroid if FEV_1 <50%

All three if symptoms/exacerbations despite these

May also have theophylline, mucolytics

Pulmonary rehabilitation

Prompt treatment for any infective exacerbation

Short course of oral steroids

Antibiotics if increased sputum purulence

Non-invasive ventilatory support for type II respiratory failure in exacerbations on maximal medical therapy

LTOT if PaO_2 <7.3 kPa when stable or <8.0 kPa with

polycythaemia/ankle oedema/pulmonary hypertension/
nocturnal desaturation – aim for at least 15 hours O_2 per day

SEQUELAE
Cor pulmonale
Bronchiectasis with recurrent infections

COMMENT

Spirometric grading of COPD

FEV$_1$/FVC	FEV$_1$	Stage
<0.7	>80% predicted	Mild (if symptomatic)
	50–79%	Moderate
	30–49%	Severe
	<30%/respiratory failure	Very severe

Identifying asthma precipitants, including a good occupational/social
history and symptom diary, is vital. Ensure good inhaler technique.

INTERSTITIAL LUNG DISEASE

Fibrotic lung diseases may be secondary to drugs or inflammation, or primary (idiopathic pulmonary fibrosis – IPF). Interstitial inflammation may be due to allergy (hypersensitivity pneumonitis), parasites (eosinophilic pneumonia), vasculitis or unknown (cryptogenic organising pneumonia – COP)

PC	**SOB**
	Dry cough – if productive, ? coexistent bronchiectasis/COP
HPC	Acute/episodic/chronic
	Exercise tolerance
	Pleuritic pain (connective tissue disease, asbestos)
	Wheeze (asthma/Churg–Strauss syndrome, sarcoid)
	Haemoptysis (? complicating infection/VTE/cancer)
PMH	Previous radiotherapy (radiation pneumonitis → fibrosis)
	Previous pneumothorax
	Asthma/rhinitis (Churg–Strauss syndrome)
	Renal disease (vasculitis/Goodpasture's syndrome)
SH	**Smoking**
	Asbestos exposure
	Occupation (pneumoconiosis in miners, farmers' lung)
	Hobbies (bird fanciers' lung)
	Travel history (TB/parasites with eosinophilic pneumonia)
DH	Amiodarone (even if well established)
	Methotrexate and many others – suspect any new drug
ROS	Constitutional symptoms (? connective tissue disease)

EXAMINATION

General appearance
Clubbing (IPF, asbestosis, hypersensitivity pneumonitis, RA)
Rheumatoid hands/nodules; scleroderma; Raynaud's
phenomenon; sicca

Respiratory
Reduced expansion (restrictive defect)
Fine fixed 'Velcro' inspiratory crackles
Bibasally in IPF (90%+), asbestosis, connective tissue
disease-associated interstitial lung disease, drug
induced
Apically in ankylosing spondylitis
Inspiratory 'squeaks' of bronchiolitis
Hypersensitivity pneumonitis, interstitial pneumonia
Expiratory wheeze due to airway inflammation
Asthma, eosinophilic pneumonia, Churg–Strauss
syndrome

INVESTIGATIONS
FBC, U&Es, LFTs
CRP/ESR
ABG – type I respiratory failure is common
Autoantibodies
Precipitins (IgG vs allergen in hypersensitivity pneumonitis)
Urinalysis
Chest radiograph – may be normal in 10%
HRCT – if typical of IPF may not need bronchoscopy
Bronchoscopy – for bronchoalveolar lavage ± biopsy
Spirometry
Restrictive (low FVC, high/normal ratio)
Reduced gas transfer factor (T_{LCO})
Six-minute walk – desaturation indicates poor prognosis

CHEST RADIOGRAPH FINDINGS

Fibrotic changes: poor expansion. Bilateral (? basal) increased density/lung markings/reticulonodular changes
Patchy 'flitting' consolidation seen with, for example, hypersensitivity pneumonitis, COP, pulmonary haemorrhage in vasculitis

TREATMENT

Stop smoking
Pulmonary rehabilitation programme
Consider supplemental oxygen (LTOT/as required)
Consider PPI (GORD may exacerbate cough)

Specific treatments depending on diagnosis:

IPF – prednisolone, azathioprine and N-acetylcysteine
COP – rule out infection; high-dose steroids
Hypersensitivity pneumonitis – avoid precipitants, ? steroids
Connective tissue disease-associated – high-dose steroids except for systemic sclerosis (risk of renal crisis)
Drug induced – withdraw drug; steroids for amiodarone

If the diagnosis is unclear – ? therapeutic trial of steroids (!)

SEQUELAE

Any of the inflammatory interstitial lung diseases can progress to fibrosis
Pulmonary hypertension
Lung cancer: 10 times increased risk, multiplicative with smoking
Pneumothorax (rare)

COMMENT

Some causes of ILD (most common first)

Idiopathic pulmonary fibrosis (cryptogenic fibrosing alveolitis)

> Histological lesion is usual interstitial pneumonia (UIP)

Sarcoidosis (case 30)

Hypersensitivity pneumonitis (extrinsic allergic alveolitis)

> Bird fanciers' lung is most common in the UK

> Farmers' lung (hay mould)

Connective tissue disease associated

> Rheumatoid arthritis (case 63)/SLE (case 64)

> Systemic sclerosis (case 68)

> Polymyositis/dermatomyositis (almost never clubbed – case 81)

Systemic vasculitis

> Wegener's granulomatosis/microscopic polyangiitis

> Churg–Strauss syndrome

Cryptogenic organising pneumonia (bronchiolitis obliterans organising pneumonia)

Pneumoconiosis – coal, silicon, beryllium, cotton

ILD associated almost exclusively in smokers

> Desquamative interstitial pneumonia

> Respiratory bronchiolitis interstitial lung disease

> Langerhans' cell histiocytosis

PNEUMONIA

Community-acquired pneumonia is a common reason for hospital admission, especially in those with underlying respiratory disease, while hospital-acquired pneumonia can complicate any admission, particularly after surgery/immobility.

PC	SOB with cough (purulent/blood-stained sputum)
	Fever, rigors, musculoskeletal aches and pains
	Acute confusion (CURB65 – see Comment)
HPC	Preceding upper respiratory tract infection
	Chest pain (pleuritic)
PMH	Asthma, COPD
	Previous chest infections
SH	Smoking
DH	Previous antibiotics; allergies
ROS	Loss of appetite, weight loss, night sweats (consider atypical/chronic infection, malignancy)

EXAMINATION

General appearance

Tachypnoea (CURB65 – see Comment)

Tachycardia, low blood pressure – ? severe sepsis (case 145)

Respiratory

Signs of collapse/consolidation:

Dullness to percussion

Increased TVF/VR

Coarse crepitations that shift with coughing

Bronchial breathing

Reduced breath sounds

Extras   Temperature chart
Sputum pot

INVESTIGATIONS

FBC	Raised WBC (neutrophilia) ± platelets (acute phase)
CRP	Raised
U&E	Urea >7.0 mmol/l (CURB65)
LFTs	Liver involvement with atypical infections
ABG	Type I respiratory failure; lactate for tissue perfusion
	Maybe type II respiratory failure if failing/COPD

Blood cultures within 6 hours, and before antibiotics
Sputum cultures, if possible with microscopy and Gram stain

CHEST RADIOGRAPH FINDINGS

Focal (? lobar) or patchy areas of consolidation ± collapse – look for the heart borders, hemidiaphragms and fissures. Air bronchograms in consolidation. Tracheal shift/volume loss if collapse. Associated parapneumonic effusion/empyema.

TREATMENT

For severe sepsis see Emergency skills (case 145)

Antibiotics guided by microbiology findings or as per local guidelines. The BTS recommends:

Outpatient:
Amoxicillin orally
Clarithromycin/doxycycline if allergic

Inpatient, low risk:
Amoxicillin + clarithromycin orally

Inpatient, high risk:
Co-amoxiclav + clarithromycin iv
Second-/third-generation cephalosporin if allergic
Switch to oral when clinical improvement occurs

A 7-day course is sufficient for low-risk patients

Oxygen: maintain SaO_2 94–98% (88–92% in CO_2 retainers)

Stop smoking

Consider immunisation against pneumococcus and influenza in at-risk individuals

SEQUELAE

Bronchiectasis, lung abscess

Pleural effusion (exudative)/empyema

Consider follow-up chest radiograph after 6 weeks if non-resolved signs or symptoms (eg chronic cough) or risk of cancer (>50, smoker)

COMMENT

The British Thoracic Society recommends risk-assessing patients with pneumonia using the CURB65 score:

Confusion of new onset (AMTS <8, see page 5)

Urea > 7.0 mmol/l

Respiratory rate > 30 breaths/min

Blood pressure 90/60 mmHg (either systolic or diastolic)

65+ years of age

CURB65 <2: consider outpatient treatment

CURB65 2: consider short inpatient stay

CURB65 >2: high risk of death, inpatient treatment ± ICU

Strep. pneumoniae (Gram positive) is the most common cause of community-acquired pneumonia in adults. The classic presentation is with lobar pneumonia, with blood-flecked 'rusty-brown' sputum.

Gram-negative infection, eg with *Haemophilus*, *Klebsiella* spp., *E. coli* or *Pseudomonas* spp., is more common in hospital inpatients, on aspiration of stomach contents or in colonising patients with chronic lung disease.

Staph. aureus infection can follow upper respiratory tract infection with influenza, and causes an aggressive necrotising pneumonia with cavitation and abscess formation, and may require combination antibiotics to cover MRSA, eg linezolid/clindamycin/rifampicin.

Mycoplasma pneumoniae can have a less acute course, and is associated with cold agglutinins and haemolytic anaemia.

Legionella pneumophila causes Legionnaires' disease and the less severe Pontiac fever when the bacteria replicate in a contaminated water source. In both cases, constitutional symptoms, fever and muscle aches are common. *Legionella* sp. is notable for many extrapulmonary symptoms in addition to a (usually bibasal) pneumonia, eg headache, confusion, diarrhoea and abnormal LFTs. *Legionella* sp. is a notifiable disease; diagnosis is with a urinary antigen test.

Viral chest infection with influenza (during epidemics), varicella-zoster (chickenpox) and cytomegalovirus (immunosuppressed patients) may give a generalised pneumonitis rather than a focal pneumonia, with a rise or fall in lymphocytes (little neutrophil response). Treatment is with specific antivirals where available.

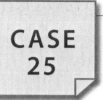

CASE 25

BRONCHIAL CARCINOMA

Lung cancer is divided histologically into small-cell (SCLC) or non-small cell lung cancer (NSCLC – squamous cell or adenocarcinoma).

PC	Thoracic	Cough (>3 weeks)/haemoptysis
		Chest/shoulder pain/stridor/hoarseness
		Breathlessness/pneumonia (esp. recurrent)

HPC   Non-specific
        Weight loss/anorexia/malaise
    Metastatic
        Back pain/bony pain (bone metastases)
        Thirst/polyuria ($\uparrow$ Ca^{2+}: bone metastases or PTH-related peptide)
        Headache (of raised ICP – 95 mmHg see Case 95)
        Hand weakness/sensory disturbance (case 73)
        Leg weakness (Lambert–Eaton myasthenic syndrome)

PMH   COPD (shares risk factors, ie smoking – case 22)
        Pulmonary fibrosis (10 times risk of adenocarcinoma – case 23)
        TB (impacts on treatment)

SH   Smoking/passive smoking
        Asbestos/chromium/nickel exposure (occupation)

ROS   Including complications of the disease and its treatment, eg nausea after chemotherapy

EXAMINATION

General appearance
        Cachectic/tachypnoeic/muscle wasting

Hands   Tar staining/clubbing (case 72)
        Hypertrophic pulmonary osteoarthropathy (HPOA)

Neck   Lymphadenopathy (case 75)

Face   Horner's syndrome (case 112)/SVCO (case 28)
Hoarse voice (recurrent laryngeal nerve palsy)

Respiratory
Pleural effusion (case 27)
Lobar collapse or consolidation (case 24)
Radiotherapy tattoos/thoracoscopic or surgical scars

Abdominal
Hepatomegaly/ascites

CNS   Papilloedema/cerebellar syndrome/neuropathy

Other   There are many non-metastatic complications of malignancy,
especially with small (oat) cell carcinoma of the lung:
Hypercalcaemia (bone metastases/PTH-related
peptide)/hyponatraemia (SIADH)/ectopic ACTH
Polyneuropathy/autonomic neuropathy
Lambert–Eaton myasthenic syndrome
Cerebellar syndrome/dementia/myelopathy
Thrombophlebitis migrans/acanthosis nigricans
Anaemia/polycythaemia

INVESTIGATIONS

FBC
U&Es
LFTs and calcium
Sputum cytology
Chest radiograph/CT of the thorax/staging CT of the chest/
abdomen/pelvis
Pleural aspiration/percutaneous biopsy
Bronchoscopy ± biopsy
Lung function (to assess fitness for surgery)
CT of the brain/ultrasonography of the abdomen/bone scan
Endocrine tests, eg serum/urine osmolality, ACTH, PTH
PET scan/surgical biopsy if no diagnosis despite the above

CHEST RADIOGRAPH FINDINGS (MAY BE NORMAL)

Discrete (often rounded) opacity with/without fibrosis

Collapse/consolidation, especially if non-resolving

Narrowing of a large bronchus

Lymphadenopathy: hilar, paratracheal

TREATMENT

NSCLC: treatment depends on staging:

Stage I/Stage II – surgery ± radiotherapy/chemotherapy

Stage IIIA – radical radiotherapy + chemotherapy

Stage IIIB – chemotherapy alone

Stage IV – symptomatic, including palliative radiotherapy

Lobectomy is preferred where possible; limited resection or CHART (continuous hyperfractionated accelerated radiotherapy) can be used in patients unsuitable for definitive surgery or chemotherapy

SCLC: treatment depends on spread – relapse is common

Within one hemithorax – radiotherapy + chemotherapy; consider prophylactic cranial irradiation

Both lungs/distal metastases – chemotherapy alone

Chemotherapy is commonly with a third-generation drug, eg docetaxel, and a platinum-based drug, eg cisplatin

Palliative radiotherapy, eg for recurrent haemoptysis, SOB, chest pain, cough, distal metastases

SEQUELAE

Common sites of metastasis:

Brain

Bone

Liver

Adrenals

COMMENT

Consider urgent referral to a lung cancer multidisciplinary team for persistent haemoptysis in a smoker aged >40 years, or anyone with SVCO or stridor (emergency referral).

Histological types

Squamous	Most common in smokers
Adenocarcinoma	Most common in non-smokers
Small (oat) cell	Fast growing, metastasise early

Simplified staging of NSCLC

I	Tumour not invading adjacent structure/>2 cm from carina; no lymph node involvement
II	Tumour as I with ipsilateral bronchial nodes
or	Tumour invading chest wall/diaphragm/mediastinal pleura/pericardium; no nodes
IIIa	Tumour as I with ipsilateral nodes including hilar/subcarinal, or II with any ipsilateral node
IIIb	Contralateral nodes (any tumour size)
or	Tumour invading heart/oesophagus/trachea/great vessels/vertebral body
or	Tumour with malignant effusion
or	Tumour with satellite nodules in same lung
IV	Metastatic disease (5-year survival rate <20%)

CASE 26   CYSTIC FIBROSIS

PC	Recurrent chest infections	
HPC	Chest	Chronic cough/sputum (volume, colour, purulence)
		Breathlessness/wheeze
		Frequency/severity of infections; admissions
		Postural drainage? Who helps with this?
		Past pneumothoraces
	GI	Weight loss/failure to thrive/constipation
		Exocrine pancreatic failure (malabsorption) in about 90%
		Jaundice (cirrhosis in about 10%)
	CVS	Cardiac failure secondary to pulmonary HTN
	Endocrine	
		Diabetes (due to pancreatic damage, about 10%)
	Other	Lethargy in hot weather due to salt loss in sweat
		Nasal polyps
		Infertility (see below)
PMH	About 10% had meconium ileus as a neonate	
	Heart–lung transplantation (case 43)	
FH	Autosomal recessive (two-thirds have ΔF508 mutation)	
	Carrier rate is around 1:25, but varies widely globally	
SH	Who assists with postural drainage/physiotherapy?	
	Problems with schooling/employment	
DH	Pancreatic enzyme supplements; insulin	
	Bronchodilators; mucolytics (eg DNAse)	
	Vitamin supplementation	
	Steroids/antibiotics for infections	

EXAMINATION

General appearance
Younger patient/short stature/decreased muscle bulk
Clubbing
Portacath for recurrent intravenous antibiotics

Respiratory
Scars from chest drains, transplantation
Cough/crackles/wheeze
Pneumothorax (case 31)

CVS   Cor pulmonale
Raised JVP/Giant 'V' waves of TR
Right ventricular heave at sternal edge
Ankle oedema

GI   Signs of chronic liver disease (cirrhosis – case 36)

INVESTIGATIONS
FBC   Anaemia/raised WBC with infection
U&Es   Salt loss
LFTs   ? Cirrhosis
Sputum (colonisation with *Haemophilus*, *Pseudomonas* spp.)
Faecal elastase for malabsorption
Lung function tests
Chest radiograph

CHEST RADIOGRAPH FINDINGS
Signs of bronchiectasis: thickened bronchi seen end-on (ring shadow) or transversely (tram track)
Signs of chronic lung disease: increased lung markings
Signs of complications: pneumothorax

TREATMENT

Physiotherapy/postural drainage
Exercise and good nutrition
Bronchodilators/mucolytics
Pancreatic enzyme/vitamin supplements
Antibiotics early and often/prophylactically
Non-invasive ventilation, eg overnight BiPAP
Heart–lung transplantation

SEQUELAE

Median life expectancy is now 38 years and rising

COMMENT

Male infertility in CF is due to the absence of the vas deferens, and consequent azoospermia. Sperm production by the testes is normal, so with assisted conception techniques reproduction is possible. Female infertility is more complex, and often related to under-nourishment and/ or thickened cervical mucus.

CASE 27

PLEURAL EFFUSION

This is an extremely common case and should be well performed.

Introduce and expose

Observe Chest movement reduced on affected side:
Cachexia/mastectomy

Hands Clubbing/tar stains
Rheumatoid hands/tendon nodules

Face Cyanosis/SLE butterfly malar rash

Neck Lymphadenopathy
Trachea deviated away from large effusion or towards effusion associated with collapse (? infection/tumour)

Chest

Inspect Radiotherapy tattoos:
Aspiration/chest drain scars/dressings

Palpate Reduced expansion on affected side

Percuss 'Stony dull' basal percussion with reduced TVF

Auscultate Decreased breath sounds/vocal resonance
May have bronchial breathing/crackles at upper limit of effusion

Extras Ankle oedema (CCF, nephrotic, liver failure, VTE)
Temperature chart/sputum (? blood stained)
Signs/risk of TB (age, ethnicity)

INVESTIGATIONS

Chest radiograph
Pleural fluid analysis – MC&S, biochemistry, cytology
Pleural biopsy (if mesothelioma suspected)
Sputum analysis – MC&S, cytology

CHEST RADIOGRAPH FINDINGS

'White out' at the base with no air bronchograms; obscures hemidiaphragm and costophrenic angle; may be a meniscus at lateral edge.

COMMENT

Pleural effusions can be classed as transudates or exudates. Differentiation based on fluid–protein level (<30 g/l = transudate, >30 g/l = exudate) is simple but inaccurate, especially in the ill patient who may have little serum protein to exude.

Light's criteria are more reliable: exudate if two or more of:

> Fluid:serum protein ratio >0.5
>
> Fluid:serum LDH ratio >0.6
>
> Fluid LDH >0.7 × lab upper limit of normal (≈200 U/l)

The same clinical and radiographic signs are given by empyema (post-pneumonia/pleural procedure), haemothorax (trauma) and chylothorax (damage to thoracic lymphatics). These are normally apparent macroscopically, but remember that empyemas are acidic relative to serum (pH <7.2).

Causes

Exudate (inflammatory)	*Transudate (hydrostatic)*
Tumour (primary/secondary)	Cardiac failure
PE/infarction	Nephrotic syndrome
Infection – pneumonia, TB	Liver failure
SLE/rheumatoid	
Subphrenic irritation (abscess, pancreatitis)	

There are many rarer causes. Mesothelioma is usually associated with clubbing and pleuritic pain, and occurs almost exclusively after asbestos exposure. Rheumatoid effusions classically have a very low glucose.

Treatment would include symptomatic drainage and treatment of the underlying condition.

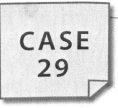

CASE 29 — OLD TUBERCULOSIS

Introduce and expose

Observe

Elderly/Asian

Abnormally shaped chest

Hands

Face

Neck   Trachea deviated to side of collapse

Chest

Inspect   Old thoracotomy scar/ribs missing/phrenic nerve crush scar

Palpate   Decreased expansion (on one side)

Percuss   Dull over area of collapse; TVF may be decreased

Auscultate

Crackles/bronchial breathing

May be fine crackles over upper lobe fibrosis

CHEST RADIOGRAPH FINDINGS

Disease: upper lobe infiltrates/cavities with fibrosis tracking to the hilum; may be hilar lymphadenopathy

Treatment: volume loss (upward-deviation of the horizontal fissure), raised hemidiaphragm (phrenic nerve crush), round air-filled ping-pong balls at apex (plombage)

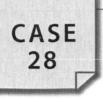
SUPERIOR VENA CAVAL OBSTRUCTION

The patient may complain of headaches/light-headedness/syncope.

Introduce and expose

Observe   Stridor/dyspnoea

Hands   Clubbed/tar stained

Face   **Oedematous**/puffy eyes
Cyanosed

Neck   **Fixed engorged neck veins (non-pulsatile JVP)**
Lymphadenopathy

Chest   Tortuous venous collaterals
Signs of chest tumour

Extras   Horner's syndrome
Radiotherapy tattoo

CHEST RADIOGRAPH FINDINGS

Discrete mass or prominence/nodularity to great vessel marking
(right paratracheal). May be signs of tracheal compression/devia
lymphadenopathy.

Causes   **Bronchial carcinoma**
Lymphoma
Retrosternal goitre/mediastinal fibrosis

COMMENT

Urgent treatment with radiotherapy or stenting is require

Tattoos are used as a fixed landmark when directing radi
they are no more than a small blue/black dot.

COMMENT

The signs are variable but are due to **fibrosis and scarring**, leaving areas without working lung tissue. The apex is most often affected but signs of apical disease can be difficult to pick up. Beware!

Complications

Fungal mycetoma in cavities, eg *Aspergillus* spp

Malignant change in old scar tissue

TB has a propensity for well-ventilated, poorly perfused areas of lung; before anti-TB drugs pneumothorax, plombage and phrenic nerve crush were all used as apical volume reduction.

Multi-drug therapy is indicated to prevent antibiotic resistance – commonly rifampicin + isoniazid for 6 months, pyrazinamide + ethambutol for the first 2 months – 'RIPE' regimen.

CASE 30 SARCOIDOSIS

Sarcoidosis is an uncommon, multisystem, non-caseating granulomatous disease of unknown aetiology, with a variable clinical presentation and severity. Symptoms include non-specific constitutional malaise, joint aches, dry eyes and breathlessness.

Introduce and expose

Observe   Tachypnoeic:
Features of thyroid disease (hypo- or hyperthyroidism)

Face   Lupus pernio, commonly nose, ears, cheeks/forehead
Red eye (uveitis)

Neck   May be lymphadenopathy

Chest

Palpate   Reduced expansion

Auscultate
Fine fixed end-expiratory crackles if fibrotic disease
Wheeze (large airway narrowing if bronchostenosis)

Extras   Erythema nodosum (especially on the shins)

INVESTIGATIONS – FOR EXTRATHORACIC DISEASE

U&Es   Renal failure

LFTs   Liver failure

Bone profile
Hypercalcaemia (due to excess vitamin D production)

TFTs   Thyroid disease

Serum ACE
High levels support the diagnosis

ECG   Arrhythmias

CHEST RADIOGRAPH FINDINGS

Bihilar lymphadenopathy, with or without reticulonodular (fibrotic) changes; scarring/bullae/cystic change in advanced disease

COMMENT

The classic clinical triad of erythema nodosum, arthralgia and bihilar lymphadenopathy, known as Löfgren's syndrome, carries a good prognosis. If treatment is required, most commonly steroids are used.

CASE 31   PNEUMOTHORAX

Spontaneous pneumothorax occurs particularly in tall, thin young men, or it may occur as a result of trauma or lung damage and increased intrathoracic pressures in COPD, asthma or infection.

Introduce and expose

Observe   Tachypnoea

Visibly reduced chest wall movement on one side

? Tall, thin/wheezy/signs of COPD (case 22)

Hands   Tar staining

Neck   Trachea pushed away from affected side (tension pneumothorax – a pre-arrest sign)

Chest

Inspect   Reduced chest wall movement unilaterally

Palpate   Reduced expansion unilaterally

Percuss   Hyperresonant over affected side:

TVF reduced

Auscultate

Reduced breath sounds over affected side

Vocal resonance high pitched

CHEST RADIOGRAPH FINDINGS

Lack of lung markings at the pleural margin, lung edge visible, separated from the pleura. The lung may be partially or completely collapsed, with increased lung markings and volume loss on that side. The size of the rim of air can be used to estimate the volume of the pneumothorax, and guide treatment.

TREATMENT

If small (<2 cm rim of air) and asymptomatic, can be managed conservatively. Otherwise needle aspiration to reinflate the lung should be attempted before considering a chest drain. If the pneumothorax persists, putting the drain on suction may be considered by a chest physician – refer for specialist advice.

For a tension pneumothorax immediate decompression with a venous cannula inserted in the second intercostal space, midclavicular line, followed by a formal chest drain, is mandatory.

OBSTRUCTIVE SLEEP APNOEA

PC	From patient: Excessive daytime sleepiness/tiredness Unrefreshing sleep/poor concentration Depression/decreased libido/nocturia From partner: Snoring/choking/witnessed apnoeas Irritability/mood change/restless sleep
HPC	Important to get a collateral history from a sleeping partner Previous treatments tried Epworth Sleepiness Score/sleep habit
PMH	Obesity/diabetes (three times risk) Hypertension (independently associated with obstructive sleep apnoea) Cardiovascular/cerebrovascular disease Respiratory/neurological (may mimic/compound effects)
FH	? Genetic influence on jaw/pharynx morphology
SH	Impact on life/work/relationships Excessive alcohol consumption/smoking
DH	Sedative drugs

EXAMINATION

General appearance

Obesity (50%) – measure height, weight and calculate BMI
Evidence of thyroid disease (case 62), acromegaly (case 59), Marfan's syndrome

BP	Large cuff if required (case 18)
Neck	Neck circumference (often >17 inches/43 cm)

Face   Mandibular/nasal deformity
Macroglossia/tonsillar hypertrophy/dentition

Respiratory
Chest wall deformities
Cor pulmonale as a complication of chronic OSA

CNS   Myopathy (case 102)/hypotonia as a cause

Legs   Ankle oedema suggesting cor pulmonale

INVESTIGATIONS

FBC   May be polycythaemic
ABG   ? Daytime hypoxia/hypercapnia
Spirometry
Polysomnography is the gold standard

CHEST RADIOGRAPH FINDINGS

Often normal

TREATMENT

Behavioural changes:
Stop smoking
Weight loss
Stop/reduce alcohol intake, sedative medications
Nocturnal continuous positive airways pressure (CPAP): this acts as a pneumatic splint, maintaining upper airway patency, using a nasal/facial mask
Intraoral devices: mainly work by anterior mandibular advancement
Surgery: tonsillectomy/nasal/mandibular surgery

COMMENT

Obstructive sleep apnoea has a structural/mechanical cause for apnoeas, as opposed to a central cause. It is generally associated with soft-tissue collapse of the airway exacerbated by decreased muscle tone, increased soft tissue or structural airway features.

Severity of obstructive sleep apnoea is based on the apnoea–hypopnoea index (AHI):

None:	<5 apnoeas/hypopnoeas per hour of sleep
Mild:	5–14 per hour
Moderate:	15–30 per hour
Severe:	>30 per hour

An apnoea is a 1-second pause in breathing associated with either neurological arousal (EEG change) or desaturation of ≥3–4%.

Important alternative diagnoses are narcolepsy and the obesity/hypoventilation or 'pickwickian' syndrome. Diagnostic criteria for this are: BMI ≥30 kg/m^2, daytime $PaCO_2$ ≥6kPa, associated sleep-related breathing disorder, no other known cause of hypoventilation.

PRESENTING A CHEST RADIOGRAPH

You may be asked to present a chest radiograph with or without a clinical history. If you have no information other than the radiograph then a systematic approach is doubly important to ensure that you miss nothing. Remember, X-rays are invisible – the film that you are looking at is a radiograph/plain film.

Technical factors

Posteroanterior (PA, usual) or anteroposterior (AP)

Adequacy of field: lungs from apex to costophrenic angles

Adequacy of exposure: vertebrae just visible behind the heart

Adequacy of inspiration: more than seven posterior or ten anterior ribs visible over lung fields

Rotation: clavicular heads equidistant from spinous process

Artefacts

Oxygen tubing

Cardiac monitoring

ET tube/tracheostomy

Chest drains:

Seldinger type pointing to apex for pneumothoraces/at base for drainage of effusion/empyema

Argyle type for trauma/haemothorax

Central venous lines: CVP lines, dialysis lines, Swann–Ganz catheter

NG tubes: crossing the diaphragm!

Pacemakers: one wire into RV (VVI), two into RA and RV (DDD), with third running outside LV (biventricular)

Sternal wires and valve prostheses

Lung borders

Blunting of costophrenic angles: pleural effusions

Loss of clear hemidiaphragms: pleural effusions, lower lobar consolidation

Raised hemidiaphragm (right usually <2 cm higher than left) indicates:

Pleural effusion

Phrenic nerve palsy/crush (treatment for TB)

Volume loss (lobar collapse, partial resection); pushed upwards (hepatomegaly, subphrenic abscess); pleural thickening

Loss of right heart border: right middle lobe consolidation

Loss of left heart border: left lingular consolidation

Hilar lymphadenopathy: bronchial carcinoma, lymphoma, sarcoidosis, chronic infection eg TB, pneumoconiosis, allergic alveolitis

Trachea and large airways

Tracheal deviation towards collapse/atelectasis, volume reduction surgery, fibrosis

Tracheal deviation away from large effusion, pneumothorax, paratracheal mass

Pleural plaques: asbestos exposure

Fluid expanding the horizontal fissure

Lung markings

Increased: pulmonary oedema, fibrosis, chronic lung disease

Opacities: dense, eg fluid; patchy, eg infection

Decreased markings: emphysema

Air bronchograms: consolidation around air-filled bronchus

Thickened bronchi: rings and tramlines with bronchiectasis

Distinct lesions: defined round opacities (malignancy), cavitating lesions (granulomatous disease, eg TB, Wegener's granulomatosis; abscesses), bullae in emphysematous COPD

Cardiovascular

Heart size and shape:

Cardiothoracic ratio (CTR) only valid on PA projection, cardiomegaly >0.5

'Globular' heart of pericardial effusion

Widened mediastinum (aortic dissection, lymphadenopathy)

Bones and soft tissue

> Rib fractures (trauma, ? pneumothorax/haemothorax)
> Vertebral collapse (osteoporosis, metastatic disease/myeloma)
> Clavicles and shoulders
> Surgical emphysema with, for example, trauma, chest drain

Review areas

If there is no abnormality so far, double-check that you have not missed anything. Commonly overlooked areas are behind the heart/apices or below the diaphragm.

COMMON DIAGNOSES

Lobar pneumonia (case 24)

Patchy/confluent opacification with air bronchograms. May be associated collapse of the lobe, which may pull the trachea towards the affected side.

> Right upper: no additional helpful signs
> Right middle: may obscure right heart border; consolidation stops at horizontal/oblique fissures
> Right lower: may obscure right hemidiaphragm; consolidation stops clearly at oblique fissure
> Left upper: lingular consolidation obscures left heart border
> Left lower: may obscure left hemidiaphragm

Pulmonary oedema (cases 3 and 146)

Increased vascular lung markings, particularly upper-lobe blood diversion. May be perihilar oedema/'bat's wings'. Even more severe is ground-glass appearance throughout the lung fields – ARDS.

Pleural effusion (case 27)

Dense opacification at the base with loss of the costophrenic angle and hemidiaphragm. There may be a meniscus at the pleural edge. Take care with supine films (effusions will not sit at the base but be behind the aerated lung field, with increased density throughout the affected side). No air bronchograms visible. A large effusion will push the trachea towards the opposite side.

COPD (case 22)

May be areas of increased lung markings or loss of lung tissue, eg bullae. Signs of hyperexpansion: hyperinflation, flattened hemidiaphragms with long 'stretched' mediastinum. Look for areas of bronchiectasis and rule out associated infection or pneumothorax.

Fibrotic lung disease (case 23)

Increased fine lung markings which may be reticular (fine line), nodular (small spots) or reticulonodular (both). May be poor inspiration (restrictive defect) or tracheal shift towards severe fibrosis. Patchy ground-glass changes, particularly at the bases.

Pneumothorax (case 31)

Loss of lung markings at the periphery of the affected lung, especially apically. The lung edge may be visible as a thin line parallel to the pleura. The trachea may be pushed away from the affected side. Look for evidence of a cause, eg rib fractures, hyperinflated lungs.

Hilar lymphadenopathy (cases 25, 29 and 30)

Rounded, lobulated opacity at the hila. Main bronchi should still be visible – look to see that they are not compressed. Look for paratracheal and mediastinal soft-tissue expansion (suggesting widespread lymphadenopathy), upper-lobe changes of TB or any discrete mass lesion in the lung fields.

Aortic dissection

Widened mediastinum. May be tracheal deviation or downward displacement of the right hilum. If aortic calcification can be seen it may have excessive soft-tissue shadowing surrounding it. The diagnosis cannot be made on chest radiograph or ECG; request a CT aortogram if symptoms suggest dissection.

Pericardial effusion (case 4)

Cardiomegaly (CTR >0.5) with a rounded 'globular' heart and loss of the left atrial window (partially obscuring left hilum). May be associated signs of heart failure (eg pulmonary oedema) or polyserositis (eg pleural effusions). Look for sternal wires suggesting recent cardiac surgery (Dressler's syndrome).

Rib metastases

Rounded low-density areas in the ribs – check posterior and anterior areas. Look for pathological fractures or callus from previous breaks. Check the other bony areas and hila, mediastinum and paratracheal areas for lymphadenopathy. Consider either bony metastases or multiple myeloma.

Volume loss

Raised hemidiaphragm on the affected side (costophrenic angle should still be clear). May be decreased lung marking on the affected side (hyperinflation of the remaining lung) or tracheal shift towards that side – not with phrenic nerve crush, because the lung is intact but underinflated due to diaphragmatic paralysis on that side.

INHALER TECHNIQUE

You may be asked to check a patient's inhaler technique, or demonstrate or teach good technique to a (mock) patient. Do not use the patient's own inhaler yourself – if no demonstration model is available, describe what you want them to do and check their understanding by getting them to show you.

Introduce yourself and **explain** what you are going to do (verbal consent).

Ask the patient to show you how they use their inhaler.

Now take them through the process step by step:

> Prepare the inhaler for use, eg cap off, shake if needed
> Take a breath in and let it out fully
> Place the inhaler in the mouth with a small gap between the inhaler and lips
> Start to breathe in through the mouth
> While breathing in, press the button to release the drug
> Continue to breathe in steadily until the lungs are full
> Hold your breath for 10 seconds (count to 10)
> Slowly exhale and take a few normal breaths (30 seconds)
> Repeat for the second 'puff'
> Replace the cap and, if a steroid inhaler, rinse the mouth

Now ask the patient to demonstrate while you talk through the steps

Finally ask the patient to perform the whole sequence without prompting

CASE 35

ARTERIAL BLOOD GAS INTERPRETATION

The ABG gives a lot of useful information, such as haemoglobin, electrolytes and glucose, in addition to the blood gases and acid–base balance. Being able to get a rapid result makes it the test of choice in an acutely ill/arrested patient.

Remember that oxygen delivery to the tissues is a function of O_2 saturations and haemoglobin concentration – the contribution of any dissolved oxygen is minimal.

OXYGENATION AND VENTILATION

Is the patient hypoxaemic?

While breathing air, a PaO_2 <8.0 kPa indicates respiratory failure.

If the patient is on supplementary oxygen, this can be harder to judge.

If so: is the patient hypercapnic/hypocapnic

If $PaCO_2$ is normal/low (appropriate hyperventilation in response to hypoxia) then there is an oxygen-exchange defect – type I respiratory failure, eg pulmonary oedema, pneumonia, PE.

If $PCaO_2$ is high (>6.0 kPa) then there is hypoventilation – type II respiratory failure, eg COPD, tiring after respiratory effort.

ACID-BASE BALANCE

What is the pH?

Remember that the pH scale is logarithmic, so small changes can indicate large abnormalities. A pH of 7.1, although 'only' 0.25 below the normal range, indicates a severe acidosis.

Acid–base disorders may be compensated in full, in part, or not at all. The body does not overcompensate – two simultaneous pathologies are more likely; therefore:

> If the pH is >7.45 the primary problem is alkalosis: is there an excess of bicarbonate (SBE >2; metabolic alkalosis), a lack of CO_2 ($PaCO_2$ <4.5 kPa; respiratory alkalosis), or both (mixed)? Is there compensation?
>
> If the pH is <7.35 the primary problem is acidosis: is there a lack of bicarbonate (SBE <−2; metabolic acidosis), an excess of CO_2 ($PaCO_2$ >6.0 kPa; respiratory acidosis), or both (mixed)? Is there compensation?
>
> In the normal range it is likely that a higher pH (7.4+) represents a primary alkalosis with respiratory compensation, and vice versa.

pH	$PaCO_2$ (kPa)	SBE	Problem
High (alkalaemic) >7.45	High >6.0	High >+2	Metabolic alkalosis (part compensated)
	Normal	High >+2	Metabolic alkalosis (not compensated)
	Low <4.5	High >+2	Mixed metabolic and respiratory alkalosis (rare)
		Normal	Not compensated (acute) respiratory alkalosis, eg hyperventilation
		Low <−2	Part compensated (long-standing) respiratory alkalosis
Normal 7.35–7.45	High >6.0	High >+2	Compensated respiratory acidosis, eg COPD Compensated metabolic alkalosis, eg vomiting
	Normal	Normal	Normal acid–base balance
	Low <4.5	Low <−2	Compensated respiratory alkalosis as above Compensated metabolic acidosis, eg AKI, DKA
Low (acidaemic) <7.35	High >6.0	High >+2	Part compensated respiratory acidosis
		Normal	Acute respiratory acidosis (not compensated)
		Low <−2	Mixed metabolic and respiratory acidosis, eg renal failure with COPD
	Normal	Low <−2	Metabolic acidosis (not compensated)
	Low <4.5	Low <−2	Metabolic acidosis (part compensated)

VIVA QUESTIONS

What are the respiratory complications of asbestos exposure?

The inhalation of asbestos fibres, which cannot be cleared by the lungs, can lead to three distinct clinical problems, which may coexist.

1. Pleural plaques or diffuse pleural thickening is often apparent on a chest radiograph as a sign of asbestos exposure, and is usually benign, although it can develop into a thoracic cage restrictive lung defect or mesothelioma.

2. Asbestosis is a fibrotic lung disease, presenting much like idiopathic pulmonary fibrosis.

3. Malignant mesothelioma of the pleura is almost exclusively seen in individuals exposed to asbestos, and has a poor prognosis (median survival of 1 year).

Symptomatic patients may be entitled to compensation, because this is an occupational lung disease in most cases.

How would you assess someone's suitability for lung cancer surgery?

Non-small cell lung cancers are best treated surgically if at an early stage (I/II). However, even patients with operable lesions may not benefit from surgery if there is a high perioperative risk, based on:

Age: no age is an absolute contraindication, but patients >80 may have increased mortality, especially if large resection is needed (eg pneumonectomy) or they have stage II disease

Cardiovascular risk: assessed by history of IHD/MI/CABG, ECG, echocardiography if a murmur is present

Lung function: patients with an FEV_1 <1.5 litres for lobectomy/wedge resection or <2 litres for pneumonectomy should have their estimated postoperative FEV_1 and transfer factor calculated to gauge risk

Other factors, eg obesity, co-morbidity, cachexia, functional status

These factors should be considered in a multidisciplinary team including a chest physician, a thoracic surgeon and an anaesthetist.

This patient has oxygen saturations of 90% on air – how would you give them supplementary oxygen?

If the patient is known to retain CO_2 then saturations of 90% are acceptable. If supplementary oxygen is required consider nasal cannulae with low-flow oxygen (1–4 litres/min), because these are often more comfortable for the patient, allow talking and eating, and dry the mouth less. The dose could be titrated upwards, using a controlled flow-rate (Venturi) facemask in need, with target saturations of 94–98%.

What causes of bronchiectasis do you know?

- Pulmonary infection (especially recurrent/chronic, eg TB): risk factors include chronic lung disease, immunodeficiency

- Pulmonary inflammation (including allergy/chemical pneumonitis)

- Ciliary dysmotility (cystic fibrosis/primary ciliary dysmotility)

What is the difference between a PA and an AP chest radiograph?

A posteroanterior film is preferred because the heart is near to the radiographic plate, reducing projection of the heart shadow over the adjacent lung fields and allowing cardiac size to be more accurately assessed. The arms can also be brought behind the plate, moving the scapulae out of the lung fields. However, the patient has to be more mobile and reasonably stable to be positioned for a posteroanterior film. With unwell patients, or with portable films taken lying down/propped up in bed, it may only be possible to take an anteroposterior film.

When would you consider a patient for oxygen therapy at home?

Patients with chronic obstructive pulmonary disease may benefit from long-term oxygen therapy (LTOT). Patients must stop smoking because there is an explosion risk. The aim is for at least 15 hours of supplemental oxygen per day, at the lowest flow rate able to keep the oxygen saturations between 90 and 92%.

Patients should be considered if they have a PaO_2 <7.3 kPa while stable (approximate sats <88%), or PaO_2 <8.0 kPa (sats <89%) with evidence of cor pulmonale (eg ankle oedema), pulmonary hypertension (eg tricuspid regurgitation), nocturnal desaturation or polycythaemia (haematocrit/ packed cell volume >55%).

ABDOMINAL SYSTEM

Examination of the abdomen

This case can cover a multitude of sins. Common cases include liver and kidney disease and haematological malignancies. The key is to look for extra-abdominal signs to indicate which system is dysfunctioning and then go on to find any abdominal signs. By the end of the examination you should be able to tie the two together.

Introduce and expose (ideally fully/'nipples to knees')

Observe

Tachypnoea	Renal failure (acidosis)
Wasting	Malabsorption/malignancy
Jaundice	Liver failure
Pigmentation	Haemochromatosis/multiple transfusions
Purpura	Hypersplenism/vasculitis
Tattoos	Risk of hepatitis
Bruising	Clotting dysfunction (liver/haem)/steroid treatment (eg transplantation) /autoimmune disease/IBD
Excoriations	Cholestasis/CKD

Hands	Palmar erythema suggests liver disease	
	Dupuytren's contracture	
		Alcohol excess/idiopathic/phenytoin

Nails	Clubbing	IBD, eg Crohn's disease/coeliac disease/ cirrhosis
	Leukonychia	Hypoalbuminaemia (liver/kidney)

Arms	AV fistula	For dialysis access (or previous scars)
	Spider naevi	Liver failure (distribution of SVC)
	Asterixis	Hepatic encephalopathy/uraemia

Face	Cushingoid	Steroid treatment
	Plethora	Polycystic kidneys (polycythaemia)
	Parotid enlargement due to vomiting (alcoholism)	

Eyes	Jaundice	
	Anaemia	
	Xanthelasma	Cholesterol/biliary cirrhosis
	Kayser–Fleisher rings of Wilson's disease	

Mouth	Ulcers	Crohn's disease/steroids
	Gum hypertrophy of transplant immunosuppression	

Neck	Lymph nodes	Malignancy (especially haematological)
	Virchow's node with upper GI tumours	
	Neck lines	Feeding line (malabsorption)
		Dialysis line
		Hickman/Portacath
		(chemotherapy)

Chest	Loss of hair	Liver failure
	Spider naevi	Liver failure (distribution of SVC)
	Gynaecomastia (liver failure/spironolactone)	

Sit the patient forward and look for scars (eg nephrectomy)/sacral oedema (low protein states)/more spider naevi.

Now lie the patient as flat as possible/comfortable, with the arms resting at the sides. Get down to the patient's level.

Abdomen
   Do not hurt the patient
   Ask if they have any tenderness before touching

Inspect Visible masses/ascites/adiposity/striae/peristalsis
      Scars of previous operations (and laparoscopy ports)
      Stomas
      Engorged veins (caput medusae vs IVC obstruction)

Palpate Systematic light palpation, then deep if non-tender

Liver	From RLQ to RUQ with border of hand
Spleen	From RLQ to LUQ with tips of fingers
Kidneys	Ballot by pressing gently from behind

Percuss Delineate size/resonance of any masses

Auscultate

Bowel sounds

Bruits over aorta (just above umbilicus), renal arteries (either side of umbilicus), liver, any masses

Roll the patient on to his or her right-hand side, feel for a spleen tip under the tenth rib and test for shifting flank dullness (ascites)

Legs		
	Oedema	Low protein states
	Bruising	Coagulopathy/steroids
	Erythema nodosum	
		IBD
	Neuropathy	Alcoholism/vitamin B_{12} deficiency

Tell the examiner 'To complete my examination I would like to examine the hernial orifices and external genitalia, perform a digital rectal examination and dipstick the urine.'

CASE 36

CHRONIC LIVER DISEASE

PC   Often non-specific: lethargy/anorexia/nausea/vague
            abdominal discomfort/ankle swelling/easy bruising
            Jaundice/pruritus

HPC   Timing – likely to have been unwell for some time
            Precipitating factors – haematemesis/melaena/infection/
            operations
            Previous admissions

PMH   Prior episodes of jaundice
            Blood transfusions/clotting factors/dialysis (hepatitis risk)
            Autoimmune diseases (chronic active hepatitis)
            COPD, especially at young age/non-smoker (α_1-antitrypsin)
            Thromboses (clotting tendency → Budd–Chiari syndrome)

FH   Treatable heritable causes, eg Wilson's disease,
            haemochromatosis

SH   Take a careful alcohol history (case 139)
            High-risk occupation: publican/travelling sales/doctor

DH   May be the cause: phenothiazines (cholestasis), amiodarone,
            methotrexate, nitrofurantoin (rarely)
            Intravenous drug use (past/present)
            Herbal/Chinese medicines

ROS   Amenorrhoea/impotence/loss of libido

EXAMINATION

Signs of chronic liver disease

Palmar erythema

Clubbing

Spider naevi (examine face, upper chest, back, both arms)

Excoriations

Anaemia

Signs of decreased oestrogen breakdown: gynaecomastia, little body hair, testicular atrophy

Usually a small, shrunken liver/hepatomegaly (case 45)

Signs of portal hypertension

Splenomegaly (case 46)

Dilated veins at portosystemic anastomoses: oesophageal/rectal varices, caput medusae

Signs of decompensation

Jaundice

Encephalopathy (asterixis/behaviour changes/confusion/drowsiness)

Fetor hepaticus

Ascites (multifactorial – case 48)

Oedema, leukonychia (low albumin synthesis)

Coagulopathy (bruising, bleeding from puncture sites)

Signs of underlying cause

Hepatitis	Tattoos, intravenous drug injection sites
Alcohol	Dupuytren's contracture, neuropathy, cerebellar signs, parotid enlargement
Wilson's disease	Kayser–Fleisher rings
Haemochromatosis	
	Pigmentation of the skin
NASH	Obesity/metabolic syndrome (case 54)
PSC	Ulcerative colitis (case 37)

Signs of treatment

Inverted Y 'Mercedes Benz' or subcostal 'rooftop' scar may represent a liver transplant.

INVESTIGATIONS

FBC   Macrocytic anaemia
Low platelets (hypersplenism)

U&Es   Hyponatraemia is common

LFTs   Especially albumin (failure of synthetic function)

Coagulation
Prolonged prothrombin time/INR

Hepatitis screen (B and C)

Ultrasonography of the abdomen – hepatic/splenic size, ascites

OGD   Varices/portal hypertensive gastropathy

Autoantibodies

ANA/AMA	Primary biliary cirrhosis
ANA/SMA/LKM	Chronic active hepatitis

Immunoglobulins

↑ IgA	Alcohol
↑ IgM	Primary biliary cirrhosis
↑ IgG	Chronic active hepatitis

Iron studies
Haemochromatosis

Copper studies
Wilson's disease

Liver biopsy

TREATMENT

Abstain from alcohol

Treat for underlying cause

Hepatitis B	Interferon, antivirals eg tenofovir
Hepatitis C	Interferon/ribavirin
Autoimmune	Steroids
Wilson's disease	Chelation with penicillamine

Treat any complications

Ascites	Diuretics/salt restriction
SBP	Antibiotics
Varices	Banding/TIPSS
Encephalopathy	Lactulose/thiamine

Referral to a specialist unit for liver transplantation

SEQUELAE

Cirrhosis of any cause increases the risk of hepatocellular carcinoma – even more so with viral hepatitis.

COMMENT

Chronic liver disease is a diagnosis that you can make at the bedside; cirrhosis is a histological diagnosis made on liver biopsy.

Coagulopathy is due to hypersplenism (low platelets) and decreased synthesis of the vitamin K-dependent clotting factors (II, VII, IX, X). Factor VII has the shortest half-life and hence the prothrombin time/INR is the first to become abnormal.

'Liver function' may be assessed in terms of synthetic function (albumin/clotting) and detoxification (encephalopathy). LFTs enable you to assess biliary obstruction (raised bilirubin/alkaline phosphatase (ALP)/γ-glutamyl transferase (GGT)) and hepatocellular damage (raised aspartate transaminase (AST)/alanine transaminase (ALT)). Remember that, in a chronically diseased cirrhotic liver, transaminases may be normal or even reduced.

TIPSS, ie transvenous intrahepatic postosystemic shunting, can relieve portal pressure but leads to blood from the gut entering the systemic circulation without metabolism in the liver (risk of encephalopathy).

INFLAMMATORY BOWEL DISEASE

Crohn's disease (CD) and ulcerative colitis (UC) are most common in White people and at northern latitudes. Age of onset is commonly in early adulthood, but diagnosis may be delayed by years/decades.

PC   CD   Diarrhoea/abdominal pain/weight loss/malaise

        UC   Diarrhoea with blood and mucus/colicky pain

HPC   Relapsing–remitting course

        Stool frequency/consistency

        Tenesmus/urgency

        Fever/constitutional symptoms (most common with CD)

        Previous operations/admissions

PMH   Ankylosing spondylitis (case 69)

FH   CD can run in families (30 times risk in siblings)

SH   CD more common in smokers/UC in non-smokers

ROS   Dry/gritty red eyes

        Arthritis/arthralgia

        Jaundice (primary sclerosing cholangitis with UC)

EXAMINATION

General appearance

    Thin/pale/febrile

Erythema nodosum/pyoderma gangrenosum

    Clubbing (rarely)

Face   Uveitis/episcleritis/conjunctivitis

        Aphthous mouth ulcers (CD/UC)

Abdomen

> Multiple laparotomy scars/enterocutaneous fistulae
> Previous stomas (CD/terminal ileostomy with UC)
> Tender inflammatory mass in RIF (terminal ileal CD)
> Distended/generally tender abdomen (UC)

INVESTIGATIONS

FBC — Anaemia/infection/inflammation (raised platelets)

U&Es — Electrolyte loss from chronic diarrhoea

LFTs/albumin

ESR/CRP

Blood and stool cultures

Abdominal radiograph/CT of the abdomen

Flexible sigmoidoscopy/full colonoscopy with biopsies

Barium meal and follow-through (CD)/enema (UC/CD)

Radiolabelled white cell scan (in severe disease if other investigations contraindicated)

ABDOMINAL RADIOGRAPH FINDINGS

UC — Dilated colon (>5.5 cm wide) – risk of toxic megacolon
Loss of haustrations in left-sided colon

CD — Small bowel dilatation in obstruction

TREATMENT

Topical treatments where possible (eg distal UC)
Systemic treatments where unwell/more proximal disease:
Salicylates (eg mesalazine)
Steroids (eg Predfoam® enemas/oral prednisolone)
Intravenous fluids, antibiotics only if septic/for surgery
Nutritional support (enteral/parenteral/elemental)
Maintenance with steroid-sparing agents, eg azathioprine

SEQUELAE

UC   Remission rates correlate with disease extent not severity. About 25% of patients with pancolitis eventually have a colectomy

Disease proximal to the splenic flexure gives an increased risk of colorectal cancer – 10% after 10 years with pancolitis

Up to 5% will develop primary sclerosing cholangitis

CD   ~75% will require surgery at some point

Obstruction due to disease/previous surgery is common

Increased risk of GI carcinoma and lymphoma

COMMENT

UC affects the large bowel in a **continuous** lesion **proximally** from rectum to caecum. The disease is classified by its extent:

Distal	Rectum (proctitis) ± sigmoid (proctosigmoiditis)
Left sided	Up to the splenic flexure
Extensive	Up to the hepatic flexure
Pancolitis	To caecum ± terminal ileum ('backwash ileitis')
Macroscopically	Red, inflamed mucosa/bleeds easily/ inflammatory 'polyps'
Microscopically	Inflammation limited to the mucosa/**crypt abscesses**

Severe UC is defined by Truelove and Witt's criteria:

More than six bloody stools per day

Fever ≥38°C

Tachycardia >100 beats/min

Hb <10 g/dl

ESR >30 mm/h

Patients should be under joint medical–surgical care. If, despite 3 days of treatment, patients still have more than eight bloody stools per day/CRP >45 mg/l then 85% will require surgery.

CD can affect any part of the GI tract **'from mouth to anus'**, with patchy lesions separated by areas of normal mucosa. Strictures and fistulae (particularly perianal fistulae) are common. The terminal ileum is most commonly affected.

Macroscopically	Thickened/narrowed bowel/cobblestone appearance/'skip' lesions
Microscopically	Inflammation involves **all** layers of the gut/ **granulomas**

ALTERED BOWEL HABIT

Any alteration from a normal bowel habit may represent underlying pathology. It is important to establish what is normal for the patient.

PC   Constipation – decreased stool frequency? Difficult to pass?
           Diarrhoea – increased stool frequency? Urgency? Soft/liquid?

HPC   Blood in the stool – on the paper, in the pan, mixed with stool
           Mucus/slime
           Fatty/yellow/difficult to flush – malabsorption
           Continence
           Abdominal pain – colicky/worse/better with defecation
           Abdominal distension/bloating
           Constitutional symptoms – weight loss/anorexia/malaise
           Diet/aggravating foods

PMH   Bowel resections (as a cause/due to underlying disease)
           Neuropathy, eg diabetes/spinal damage, eg trauma/MS –
           abdominal/pelvic radiotherapy

FH   Colorectal carcinoma (eg familial adenomatous polyposis)

SH   Foreign travel/has anyone else at home been unwell?

DH   Laxatives/antidiarrhoeals
           Opiates/iron/anticholinergics, eg tricyclic antidepressants –
           constipation

EXAMINATION

General appearance

Cachexia	Malignancy/malabsorption/malnourished
Pallor	Iron deficiency/vitamin malabsorption
Clubbing	IBD/coeliac disease
Mouth ulcers	IBD/coeliac disease

Abdomen

Scars, eg reversed stomas, laparotomies (adhesions)

Abdominal distension with hyperresonance ('tympanic')

Masses – tumour, inflammatory (eg Crohn's disease), stool

Say that you would do a **digital rectal examination** (case 50)

INVESTIGATIONS

FBC Anaemic – microcytic/macrocytic/mixed

U&Es/LFTs/Ca^{2+}/TFTs

Vitamin B$_{12}$/folate/ferritin

Abdominal radiograph/barium follow-through/meal

Sigmoidoscopy/colonoscopy/OGD and duodenal biopsy

Stools for MC&S/occult blood/fat/elastase

Anti-endomysial/anti-gliadin antibodies – coeliac disease

TREATMENT

Dietary advice/laxatives/antidiarrhoeals (loperamide)

Treatment directed to underlying cause (eg antibiotics)

Irritable bowel – antispasmodics (eg mebeverine)

Autonomic neuropathy – motility stimulants (eg domperidone)

Coeliac – gluten-free diet

COMMENT

Causes of diarrhoea:

    Infective

    IBD (case 37)

    Radiation enteritis

    Malabsorption (biliary/pancreatic disease, coeliac)

    Small bowel tumours (adenocarcinoma/lymphoma/carcinoid)

    Bowel resection (short bowel/bacterial overgrowth/colectomy)

    Overflow with constipation

    Irritable bowel

    Drugs/laxative abuse/eating disorders (case 138)

    Autonomic neuropathy (eg diabetes)

    Thyrotoxicosis/hypocalcaemia

Causes of constipation:

    Poor diet/painful defecation (eg anal fissure)

    Immobility

    Large bowel tumours

    Abdominal surgery (adhesions)/ileus (eg hypokalaemia)

    Irritable bowel

    Drugs/eating disorders (case 138)

    Autonomic neuropathy (eg diabetes)/spinal cord disease

    Hypothyroidism/hypercalcaemia

CASE 39

UPPER GASTROINTESTINAL BLEED

Upper GI bleeding is commonly due to peptic ulceration, eg associated with *Helicobacter pylori*/NSAIDs/steroids, portal hypertension (varices/gastropathy), malignancy or vascular malformations (angiodysplasia/Dieulafoy's lesions)

PC
Haematemesis (fresh/altered 'coffee-ground' blood)
Melaena (black, tarry stools)
Collapse/syncope/symptomatic anaemia (case 40)

HPC
Indigestion/acid reflux/waterbrash/bloating
Pain related to (gastric)/relieved by (duodenal) eating
Anorexia/weight loss
Fatigue/decreasing exercise tolerance (anaemia)

PMH
Previous peptic ulcers/gastro-oesophageal reflux
Chronic pain (NSAIDs)
Autoimmune disease (steroids)
Chronic liver disease (portal hypertension)
Recent/current hospital admission (physiological stress)

FH
Hereditary haemorrhagic telangiectasia (case 90)

SH
Smoking, alcohol use (increased risk with *H. pylori*)

DH
Ask specifically about over-the-counter medicines (NSAIDs)
Anticoagulation (increased risk of severe bleed)
Drugs increasing risk (SSRIs)/treating (PPIs/H_2-receptor blockers)

EXAMINATION

General appearance

Pallor/tachycardia (anaemia)

Signs of shock – medical emergency

Telangiectasia

Check for a Virchow's node in the left supraclavicular fossa

Abdomen

Epigastric tenderness

Signs of chronic liver disease/portal hypertension (case 36)

INVESTIGATIONS

FBC   Microcytic anaemia (iron deficiency)

U&Es   Urea raised out of proportion to creatinine (urea in mmol/l, usually <10% of creatinine in μmol/l)

LFTs

Coagulation

Blood group and save

OGD   Diagnostic and therapeutic

H. pylori testing, eg CLO test at OGD or breath test

Capsule endoscopy to see lesions inaccessible to fibreoptic endoscopy, eg small bowel angiodysplasia

TREATMENT

Resuscitation: ABCDE approach (see Emergency skills)

Stop causative drugs, eg NSAIDs; reverse warfarin

OGD and dual/triple therapy (eg sclerotherapy with adrenaline ± cautery ± clipping)

Sengstaken–Blakemore tube for variceal haemorrhage

PPIs: intravenous omeprazole for 72 h post-endoscopic treatment reduces re-bleed risk

Ongoing antacid treatment with PPI/H_2-receptor antagonist

H. pylori eradication (PPI + two antibiotics)

SEQUELAE

May require follow-up endoscopy to assess healing

COMMENT

The Rockall score uses age, co-morbidities, haemodynamic status and findings at endoscopy to risk stratify patients:

Age (years)		Shock	
<60	0	No shock	0
60–79	1	Tachycardia	1
80+	2	Systolic BP <100 mmHg	2

Diagnosis at OGD		Bleeding	
Mallory–Weiss tear	0	No evidence	0
GI malignancy	2	Blood/clot/spurting vessel	2
All other diagnoses	1		

Co-morbidity

None	0
CCF, IHD, other major co-morbidity	2
Renal/liver failure, metastatic cancer	3

A score of ≤2 has about a 5% re-bleed risk and about a 0% mortality rate.

A score of ≥8 has about a 40% re-bleed risk and about a 40% mortality rate.

ANAEMIA

The patient may be found to be anaemic on routine testing, or have symptoms. The key to the cause is in the history.

PC	**Tired all the time** ('TATT')/lethargy/malaise
	Decreased exercise tolerance/exertional angina
HPC	Overt blood loss (stools/vomitus/urine/gynaecological)
	Covert blood loss (indigestion/altered bowel habit)
	Vitamin deficiencies (malabsorption/diarrhoea)
	Symptoms suggesting malignancy (anorexia/weight loss)
	including 'B' symptoms (fever/night sweats)
PMH	Chronic disease – infection, autoimmune, liver, kidney
FH	Hereditary haemoglobinopathies/red cell disorders
	Bleeding disorders, eg haemophilia/HHT (case 90)
SH	Diet/alcohol
	Smoking (risk of cancer)
DH	Anticoagulants/NSAIDs/steroids
ROS	Biliary colic (gallstones with persistent haemolysis)

EXAMINATION

General appearance

Pallor (most easily seen in the conjunctiva/nail beds)

Jaundice (haemolysis/chronic liver disease – case 36)

Pigmented skin from secondary haemochromatosis with multiple blood transfusions

Koilonychia ('spoon-shaped' nails of iron deficiency)

Angular stomatitis/smooth red/'beefy' tongue

Telangiectasia (case 90)

Lymphadenopathy

CVS Tachycardia

Rarely, high-output cardiac failure (case 3)

Abdomen

Hepatomegaly/splenomegaly ('honorary lymph nodes')

INVESTIGATIONS

FBC Hb, MCV, RDW, other blood cell lineages

U&Es Anaemia of CKD (case 42)

LFTs Bilirubin raised in haemolysis

CRP/ESR (anaemia of chronic disease)

Blood film

Reticulocytes

Haptoglobins (reduced), LDH (increased) – haemolysis

Hb electrophoresis – sickle cell disease/thalassaemia

Bone marrow biopsy

TREATMENT

Blood transfusion if severe/symptomatic (eg angina)

Replace vitamin/mineral deficiencies

Erythropoiesis-stimulating agents (CKD/haematological)

COMMENT

Anaemia can be classified by red cell indices (MCV, RDW):

Microcytic   Iron deficiency, thalassaemia, lead, sideroblastic anaemia, chronic disease (more often normocytic)

Normocytic   Acute haemorrhage/haemolysis, chronic disease, ↓ red cell production (eg bone marrow failure)

Mixed microcytic and macrocytic (with high RDW), eg iron deficiency and reticulocytosis with haemolysis (average cell size is still normal)

Macrocytic   Vitamin B_{12}/folate deficiency/drugs affecting DNA synthesis (eg methotrexate)/hypothyroidism/ reticulocytes

The blood film can give additional clues as to a cause, eg leukaemia, microangiopathic haemolytic anaemia (MAHA), sickle cell disease.

Haemolytic anaemia may be intravascular (dark urine) or extravascular:

Congenital   Glucose-6-phospate dehydrogenase (G6PD) deficiency/spherocytosis/sickle cell

Mechanical   Prosthetic heart valves/MAHA

Acquired   Autoimmune (primary/in combination with eg haematological malignancy, *Mycoplasma* spp.)

ACUTE KIDNEY INJURY

Any newly diagnosed renal failure should be considered acute until proven otherwise. Causes can be divided into pre-, post- and renal.

PC   **Often none/incidental finding on blood tests**
Decreased urine output
Haematuria/haemoptysis (vasculitis/Goodpasture's syndrome)

HPC   Symptoms of uraemia – GI upset/drowsiness/tremor
Symptoms of acidosis – SOB
Symptoms of fluid overload if oliguric/anuric
Thirst/diarrhoea/vomiting (dehydration)
Lower urinary tract symptoms (obstruction)
Fever/rash/joint pain/swelling (interstitial nephritis/vasculitis)

PMH   Diabetes/hypertension/CCF/CKD (predispose to AKI)
Current/previous malignancy (chemotherapy/radiation fibrosis/tumour lysis/myeloma)

DH   Drugs affecting the renin–angiotensin system (eg ACE inhibitors)
NSAIDs
Antibiotics/PPIs/any new drugs (interstitial nephritis)

EXAMINATION

General appearance

Well/unwell

Tachypnoea	Acidosis/pulmonary oedema
Asterixis	Uraemia
JVP/BP	For fluid status

CVS Pericardial rub Uraemia

Respiratory

Bibasal crepitations	Pulmonary oedema
Patchy crepitations	Infection/pulmonary haemorrhage

Abdominal

Scars/renal masses/palpable bladder

Dipstick the urine Blood/protein suggest renal cause

Legs Peripheral oedema Fluid overload/nephrotic syndrome

Purpuric rash Vasculitis

INVESTIGATIONS

FBC/U&Es/LFTs

CK rhabdomyolysis (eg after fall/poisoning/statins)

CRP/ESR

ANA (SLE), ANCA (vasculitis), anti-GBM (Goodpasture's syndrome)

Immunoglobulins and electrophoresis; cryoglobulins

ABG Degree of acidosis, rapid assessment of electrolytes

Chest radiograph To show pulmonary oedema/haemorrhage

Ultrasonography of the renal tract for renal size/obstruction

Renal biopsy

TREATMENT

For treatment of life-threatening hyperkalaemia, see case 148
Fluid resuscitation – don't overfill an anuric patient
Urine output monitoring – catheterise if necessary
Relieve obstruction – catheter/nephrostomies
Stop any toxic/exacerbating/new drugs
Early specialist opinion if suggestion of renal cause/
approaching need for dialysis (unmanageable hyperkalaemia/
acidosis/uraemia/fluid overload)

COMMENT

Prerenal

Systemic hypoperfusion	Shock, sepsis
Renal hypoperfusion	Renovascular disease, hepatic failure
Renal haemodynamics	NSAIDs, ACE inhibitors

Renal

Toxic	Gentamicin, urate, rhabdomyolysis, MAHA, contrast
Allergic	Interstitial nephritis
Autoimmune	Vasculitis

Postrenal

Supracystic obstruction	Must be bilateral, eg stones, malignancy
Bladder outflow	Prostatic, motility

Often patients have a combination of factors, eg chronic prostatic
obstruction with associated urinary tract infection leading to septic shock
while on an ACE inhibitor for underlying diabetes mellitus.

CHRONIC KIDNEY DISEASE

Think of CKD as a multisystem disorder. Patients may move through a variety of renal replacement modalities over time, eg dialysis, transplantation, fails, dialysis.

PC
Reason for admission
New diagnosis of CKD-/dialysis-related problem/complication

HPC
When was renal failure first diagnosed?
Cause of renal failure? On dialysis? How long?
Peritoneal dialysis (PD):
> Machine overnight (automated PD)?
> Manual exchanges (continuous ambulatory PD)?
> What bags do they use (often known by their colour)
> Any episodes of PD peritonitis?

Haemodialysis (HD):
> Hospital/satellite centre/home
> Vascular access (past and present) – fistula/line

Transplant – functioning/failed
Lethargy/fatigue/anorexia/GI upset/pruritus

PMH
Diabetes/hypertension
Cardiovascular disease: IHD/TIAs/CVA/claudication
Bone disease/calcium phosphate/parathyroidectomy

FH
Many genetic causes (eg polycystic kidneys/Alport's syndrome)

SH
Home alterations if home therapy – does anyone help?
Smoking
Dietary and fluid restrictions

DH
Erythropoiesis-stimulating agents (subcutaneous injection)
Phosphate binders (tablets taken with meals)
Antihypertensives
Immunosuppression (transplant/vasculitis)

ROS   Does the patient pass urine? How much?

Bowel habit is important with PD

EXAMINATION

General appearance

Pallor	Anaemia
Excoriations	Pruritus is multifactorial
Bruising	Bleeding tendency/steroids
Hearing aid	Sensorineural deafness in Alport's syndrome
Neck lines	Tunnelled across front of chest/old scars
AV fistula	Usually forearm (radiocephalic) or upper arm

CVS   BP/JVP   Hypertension/assessment of fluid status

Heaving apex/loud second heart sound

Abdominal

Scars   Transplant in iliac fossa/nephrectomy

Polycystic kidneys

Tenckhoff catheter

Check exit site (lateral to the umbilicus)

CNS   Fundi   Diabetic/hypertensive retinopathy

Peripheral neuropathy

Legs   Peripheral oedema

Urinalysis if the patient still passes urine

INVESTIGATIONS

FBC   Normocytic anaemia is common even on treatment

U&Es   The eGFR is calculated from creatinine and hence is not meaningful in dialysis patients

Calcium/phosphate/ALP/parathyroid hormone

Urinary protein:creatinine ratio

Measure of proteinuria

Ultrasonography of the renal tract

Usually small kidneys (except diabetes)

Renal biopsy if no diagnosis/kidneys not too small

TREATMENT

Lifestyle advice – stop smoking, maintain a healthy weight

Low-potassium diet (no bananas/fruit juice/chocolate)

Low-phosphate diet (minimal dairy/offal/red meat)

Fluid restriction if anuric/oliguric

Drugs

Antihypertensives (ACE inhibitors preferred if proteinuric)

Phosphate binders (eg calcium carbonate)

Activated vitamin D (eg 1-alfacalcidol)

Iron supplements (orally/intravenously)

Erythropoiesis-stimulating agents for anaemia

Immunisations: viral hepatitis, seasonal influenza

Dialysis by PD or HD is equally effective

PD removes fluid and solutes by osmosis. The dialysate can be varied in terms of osmolality (weak–strong) and solute (glucose/polymer/amino acids). PD peritonitis usually manifests itself as a 'cloudy bag' and is treated with intraperitoneal antibiotics.

HD usually requires 4 hours three times a week, although hours and frequency can be increased in patients dialysing at home. It requires good, reliable vascular access – a fistula is preferable to a plastic line.

Transplantation requires less disruption to a patient's life but involves long-term immunosuppression to prevent graft rejection, giving an increased risk of infection/malignancy. Kidneys may be obtained from deceased donors or donated by a family member or friend, but there is a great shortage.

SEQUELAE

Cardiovascular disease
> CKD is a strong independent risk factor for all forms of vascular disease

Mineral bone disease
> Hyperparathyroidism and vitamin D deficiency lead to low-/high-/mixed-turnover bone disease

Neuropathy can affect any part of the nervous system (peripheral/autonomic neuropathy/cognition)

Complications of immunosuppression
> Infection, especially opportunistic/viral reactivation
> Malignancy, especially skin cancers/lymphoma
> New-onset diabetes after transplantation

COMMENT

The most common causes of CKD requiring dialysis in the UK are:

Diabetes mellitus

Hypertension

Glomerulonephritis

Genetic kidney diseases, eg polycystic kidneys

SOLID ORGAN TRANSPLANT

You may suspect a transplant has been received if there is a surgical scar, evidence of immunosuppression or signs of an underlying disease/organ dysfunction.

Heart	Cardiomyopathy
Heart–lung	Congenital/pulmonary HTN/CF
Lung	COPD/interstitial lung disease/CF
Liver	Chronic liver disease/paracetamol
Kidney	Chronic kidney disease
Kidney–pancreas	
	Type 1 diabetes with nephropathy
Pancreas alone	
	Type 1 diabetes with hypoglycaemia

In addition to systems examination

Signs of immunosuppression

>   Skin lesions (warts, keratoses, BCCs)/excision scars
>   Mouth ulcers
>   Bruising/steroidal skin/cushingoid (steroids)
>   Gingival hypertrophy (ciclosporin)
>   Hirsutism (ciclosporin)

Complications of immunosuppression

>   Lymphoproliferative disease (EBV reactivation)
>   New-onset diabetes after transplantation
>   Tremor (calcineurin inhibitors)
>   Hypertension (calcineurin inhibitors)
>   CKD (calcineurin inhibitors)
>   Bone marrow suppression (anti-proliferatives)

COMMENT

Common immunosuppressive regimens consist of:

> Steroids (prednisolone)
>
> Calcineurin inhibitors (ciclosporin/tacrolimus)
>
> Antiproliferatives (azathioprine/mycophenolate)

Patients may be given prophylaxis against opportunistic infections such as *Pneumocystis jirovecii* (co-trimoxazole), viral reactivation/infection with donor CMV (valganciclovir), or to prevent chest infection in lung transplant recipients (azithromycin).

NEPHROTIC SYNDROME

This may be due to a primary/secondary renal disorder, or secondary to drugs/amyloid (myeloma/chronic inflammation).

PC	Swollen ankles/legs/puffy face in the morning
	Frothy urine
HPC	The nephrotic syndrome is made up of the classic triad of proteinuria/hypoalbuminaemia/oedema, with hypercholesterolaemia and hypercoagulability
	Oedema may be the only symptom
	Incidental finding on blood/urine testing
	Found during investigation for VTE (case 5)
	Ask specifically about haematuria/preceding symptoms
PMH	Diabetes
	Known malignancy/Hodgkin's lymphoma/myeloma
	Autoimmune connective tissue disease (RA/SLE)
	Chronic infections (TB, osteomyelitis, bronchiectasis)
FH	Familial kidney disease
DH	NSAID use
	Penicillamine/gold (RA)
	Captopril (cause)/other ACE inhibitors/ARBs (treatment)

EXAMINATION

General appearance
    Leukonychia (if long-standing hypoalbuminaemia)

Face   Facial/periorbital oedema
    Butterfly rash of SLE/xanthelasma of high cholesterol

CVS   Hypertension (salt and water overload)/hypotension

Respiratory
    Pleural effusions

Abdominal
    Ascites (case 48)
    Hepatomegaly/splenomegaly/both (amyloid)

CNS   Fundi
    Diabetic/hypertensive retinopathy
    Peripheral neuropathy (diabetes/HTN/SLE)

Legs   Peripheral oedema (may include sacral/abdominal oedema)

Urinalysis for heavy proteinuria ± haematuria

INVESTIGATIONS

Urinary protein:creatinine ratio – quantify proteinuria
U&Es – renal failure: volume depletion/underlying disease
LFTs – albumin often very low (<20)
Cholesterol often very high (total cholesterol >10)
Autoantibodies – rheumatoid factor, ANA, dsDNA, ANCA
Complement components (C3, C4)
Immunoglobulins and protein electrophoresis/light chains
Hepatitis/HIV/syphilis serology
Ultrasonography of the renal tract – usually normal-sized kidneys
Renal biopsy is usually necessary

TREATMENT

Diuretics/fluid restriction/salt restriction

ACE inhibitors/ARBs reduce protein loss and treat hypertension

Treat hypercholesterolaemia

Withdraw any causative drugs

Consider prophylaxis for thromboembolism

Definitive treatment depends on histological diagnosis:

Minimal change	Usually steroid responsive
Membranous	Can spontaneously remit or steroids/cyclophosphamide
Focal segmental glomerulosclerosis (FSGS)	May be slowly steroid responsive
Amyloid	Depends on underlying cause

COMMENT

Remember primary nephrotic syndrome as the disease of 3s:

Proteinuria of >3 g/day (protein:creatinine >300 mg/mmol)

A third of adults have minimal change disease

A third have FSGS

A third have membranous nephropathy, of whom:

A third spontaneously remit

A third remain nephrotic with stable disease

A third progress to end-stage renal failure

CASE 45

HEPATOMEGALY

Introduce and expose

Look for signs of chronic liver disease (case 36)

Inspect Distension in the right hypochondrium:

Striae Chronic liver disease/obesity

Scars Previous tumours (? liver metastases)

Transplants/shunts

Ascites

Stoma Primary sclerosing cholangitis with UC

Bowel tumours (? liver metastases)

Palpate Start at RIF and move up with the edge of the hand

Describe the liver edge:

Smooth Hepatitis/CCF/normal/displaced downwards (COPD)

Nodular Cirrhosis/tumour/metastases

Pulsatile Tricuspid regurgitation

Tender Hepatitis/CCF

Percussion

Upper and lower borders, measure size in mid-clavicular line (normal = 12 cm)

Check for shifting dullness if you suspect ascites

Auscultate

Bruit Hepatocellular carcinoma in cirrhosis

Arteriovenous malformation

Tricuspid regurgitation (systolic murmur at LLSE)

Don't forget the rest of the abdomen.

At the end of the case you should be able to tell the examiner 'There is isolated hepatomegaly with/without decompensated liver function'. You should comment on features that will lead you to a more definitive diagnosis.

COMMENT

Remember that the liver is a mass in the RUQ, which is dull to percussion and contiguous with the area of expected hepatic dullness, enlarges towards the RIF, moves downwards towards the RIF on inspiration and which you can't get above.

Causes   **Carcinoma** (metastatic/hepatocellular)

Cirrhosis

CCF (check JVP, ankle oedema)

Fatty liver (alcohol/non-alcoholic steatohepatitis + metabolic syndrome)

Alcoholic hepatitis

Viral infection (hepatitis/EBV/CMV/HIV)

Tropical infection (hydatid/malaria/*Leptospira* spp.)

Biliary obstruction

Myeloproliferative/lymphoproliferative disease
Infiltration (amyloid, sarcoid)

Haemoglobinopathies (eg sickle cell disease with small infarcted spleen)

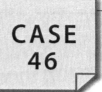

CASE 46

SPLENOMEGALY

Introduce and expose

    Look for signs of chronic liver disease (case 36)

Inspect   Swelling/bruising/purpura/petechiae

    Caput medusae (portal hypertension)

Palpate   Start at RIF and move up with the tips of the fingers

    Note the edge and notch

Percussion

    Dullness up to ninth rib/midaxillary line

    Check for shifting dullness if you suspect ascites

Auscultate

    Feel for other lymph nodes (cervical/axillary/inguinal, etc)

Don't forget the rest of the abdomen

COMMENT

Remember that the spleen is a mass in the LUQ, which is dull to percussion and contiguous with the area of expected splenic dullness, has a notch, enlarges diagonally towards the RIF, moves downwards towards the LIF on inspiration and which you can't get above.

Causes

Myeloproliferative disease

Chronic myeloid leukaemia

Myelofibrosis

Lymphoproliferative disease

Chronic lymphocytic leukaemia

Lymphoma, other leukaemias

Portal hypertension with shrunken liver

Cirrhosis

Budd–Chiari syndrome (hepatic venous occlusion)

Infection

Viral (EBV/CMV/HIV/mumps)

Bacterial (eg infective endocarditis)

Tropical (malaria, kala-azar, *Schistosoma* spp.)

Infiltration (amyloid, sarcoid)

Hyperfunction (haemoglobinopathies)

Rheumatoid arthritis (Still's disease)

HEPATOSPLENO-MEGALY

You must go over all the points covered in isolated hepatomegaly and splenomegaly. It may be difficult to distinguish between massive hepatic enlargement and hepatosplenomegaly. Check to see if the splenic dullness behind the ninth rib continues over the abdomen; if not it is more likely to be hepatomegaly alone.

Causes

Myeloproliferative disease (extramedullary haematopoiesis)

Lymphoproliferative disease (? other lymph nodes)

Cirrhosis with portal hypertension

Haemoglobinopathies (thalassaemia/sickle cell disease)

Viral infection (hepatitis/EBV/CMV/HIV)

Tropical infection (malaria/leishmaniasis (kala-azar))

ASCITES

This may appear as part of chronic liver disease or in isolation.

Introduce and expose

Inspect Swelling/everted umbilicus/vein distension

Palpate May be tense (difficult to feel organs)
Fluctuation/fluid thrill

Percussion
Stony dullness in the flanks that shifts on movement

Auscultate

Causes Chronic liver disease, especially with portal hypertension
Intra-abdominal/pelvic malignancy/liver metastases
Right-sided heart failure
Nephrotic syndrome and low-protein states
Infection, eg TB
Polyserositis, eg SLE, rheumatoid arthritis
Pancreatitis

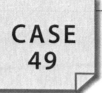

CASE 49

RENAL MASSES

There are three main possibilities:
1. **Unilateral** enlargement
2. **Bilateral** enlargement
3. **Transplanted** kidney

The extra-abdominal signs should be noted before examining the abdomen.

Introduce and expose

Look for signs of CKD

Inspect Scars in loin/transplant in groin

Palpate Bimanual palpation of mass in loin (ballotting)

Percussion Usually resonant (due to overlying bowel gas)

Auscultate Bruit Tumour/(transplant) renal artery stenosis

COMMENT

Remember a kidney is a mass in the flank that is resonant to percussion, moves downwards on inspiration, you can get above and is ballottable. The right kidney is often the easiest to feel due to downward displacement by the liver.

Causes

Normal kidneys in a thin person

Autosomal-dominant polycystic kidney disease (ADPKD) (only one kidney may be palpable)

Large renal cyst

Malignancy

Massive hydronephrosis

Hypertrophy of a single functioning kidney

Autosomal-dominant polycystic kidney disease (ADPKD) is associated with cysts in many other organs, especially the liver, spleen and pancreas. Intracranial aneurysms can be found in about 10% of patients, and risk of subarachnoid haemorrhage is increased if there is a family history of haemorrhage/sudden death or uncontrolled hypertension. Other associations are aortic root dilatation and mitral valve prolapse. Renal function declines with time, but not all patients progress to end-stage renal failure or develop the anaemia of CKD.

DIGITAL RECTAL EXAMINATION

This is now commonly performed on a model. Remember to interact as you would with a real patient – your communication skills are as important as your clinical skills.

Introduce and explain (verbal consent)

Ask for another staff member to be present as a chaperone

Wash your hands and put on gloves

Position the patient lying flat, on his left side with knees drawn up, and position the equipment close to hand

Inspect the perineum, buttocks and anus. Comment on skin tags, haemorrhoids, fissures, fistulae, etc

Lubricate your finger

Gently introduce you finger into the anal canal and rectum:

> Start with the palmar surface of the finger towards the sacrum
> Comment on any masses, internal haemorrhoids, hard stool

360° sweep of the rectum with your finger:

> Rotate your hand so that the palmar surface is uppermost
> Then sweep around until palpating the anterior part of the rectum
> Feel for the prostate – the central sulcus should be palpable
> Comment on size, symmetry and surface of the prostate

Remove your finger and examine the glove. Comment on stool colour/ presence of blood/mucus

Clean the patient, thank him and ask him to get dressed

Wash your hands and tidy your equipment

Document your findings

PASSING A NASOGASTRIC TUBE

There are two types in common use:

1 Wide-bore (Ryles) tubes for decompression of the stomach
2 Fine-bore feeding tubes for enteral feeding

The procedure is the same in both cases.

Introduce and explain (verbal consent)
Outline risks and benefits; say that insertion may be uncomfortable

Wash your hands and put on gloves

Position the patient sitting upright and have **the equipment** close to hand

Estimate the length required: nostril to earlobe (nasopharynx) + earlobe to below diaphragm

Check the nostrils for obvious deformities/septal deviation. Decide which side you wish to use (can be either)

Lubricate the tube

Pass the tube – remember that the nasopharynx extends backwards towards the occiput, not upwards

Ask the patient to swallow as he or she feels the tube in the back of the throat; advance tube to the previously estimated length. **If the patient coughs at any point, stop and reposition**

Secure the tube – consider the patient's comfort, oxygen masks, etc

Check position

Visual check of the mouth/pharynx
Fine-bore tubes checked with chest radiograph
Ryles tubes require pH check

Document the procedure in the notes and thank the patient

URINE DISPSTICK TESTING

To test the urine a fresh, clean-catch sample (mid-stream urine) or catheter specimen should be placed in an aliquot deep enough for the testing strip.

Examine the urine macroscopically and comment on colour

Place some paper towels on a flat surface

Place the test strip in the urine and start the timer

Remove the test strip, allow any excess urine to drain off

Place the test strip on the paper towel ready to be read

Read the strip as the time allotted for each reagent square to fully react is reached (up to 60 s)

Record the results and tidy up your equipment

Various dipsticks are available. Commonly you will have:

Specific gravity

High in dehydration, low with dilute urine

pH   Failure to acidify urine: tubular acidosis

Alkaline with urease-positive UTI

Leukocyte esterase

Presence of neutrophils, eg infection

Nitrites   Only positive with urease-forming bacteria (usually Gram negative)

Protein   Reagent reacts to albumin, and will miss Bence Jones and microalbuminuria – special test strips are available

Glucose   Diabetes mellitus/renal glycosuria

Ketones   Diabetic ketoacidosis

Bilirubin/urobilin

Jaundice/haemolysis

Blood   Reagent reacts to globin, hence also positive with haemolysis, myoglobinuria (rhabdomyolysis) – microscopy for red cells can help distinguish these
Intact red cells can give a 'spotty' pattern

VIVA QUESTIONS

How would you diagnose and treat Wilson's disease?

Wilson's disease (hepatolenticular degeneration) is an autosomal recessive disorder in which copper cannot be excreted into the bile by the liver. Copper accumulates in the tissues, leading to chronic liver disease (hepato-) and damage to the basal ganglia (lenticular). Symptoms include those of chronic liver disease, parkinsonism and other movement disorders (ataxia, dystonias). More rarely, heart failure (cardiomyopathy), proximal renal tubular acidosis and endocrine disorders such as hypoparathyroidism can occur.

Diagnosis might be suggested by a physical examination revealing Kayser–Fleischer rings around the iris, and confirmed with serum ceruloplasmin (low), urinary copper excretion (high), or liver biopsy. Treatment is with chelating agents such as penicillamine. Advanced liver disease is treated by liver transplantation.

What can you tell me about coeliac disease?

Coeliac disease (gluten enteropathy) is an autoimmune disease characterised by intolerance of wheat and other cereals containing gluten. Inflammation of the small bowel on exposure to gluten leads to villous atrophy (seen on duodenal biopsy) and malabsorption. Symptoms include abdominal cramping, steatorrhoea, anaemia/vitamin deficiencies, weight loss/failure to thrive and mouth ulcers. It is associated with clubbing, dermatitis herpetiformis and carcinomas/lymphomas of the small bowel. Diagnosis is made with specific autoantibodies (anti-endomysial/anti-gliadin) or duodenal biopsy. Treatment is with dietary gluten restriction.

What would you tell a patient whom you suspect has irritable bowel syndrome?

Irritable bowel syndrome is a diagnosis of exclusion – other GI disorders should be excluded before the diagnosis is made. Patients should be advised to pay attention to their diet, keeping regular mealtimes, drinking plenty of fluid while restricting caffeine and alcohol, and reducing foods high in insoluble fibre. Soluble fibre (oats/ispaghula) may help, as may anti-spasmodics (mebeverine).

What problems does sickle cell disease cause?

Sickle cell disease, due to the presence of haemoglobin SS (HbSS), can lead to a number of acute and chronic complications. Painful (vaso-occlusive) crises can occur when low oxygen tension leads to 'sickling' of the red blood cells, which become inelastic and block small blood vessels, leading to end-organ ischaemia. These require oxygen and often high-dose opiate analgesia. Common sites are the extremities (dactylitis, priapism), bones (avascular necrosis) and spleen, although any organ can be affected. Chronic damage to the spleen leads to autosplenectomy and risk of infection with encapsulated organisms (eg pneumococci). Shorter red cell lifespan leads to susceptibility to aplastic anaemia with parvovirus B19 infection. Excess haemoglobin turnover can lead to gallstones.

What are the complications of blood transfusion?

Transfusion reactions include fever at the time of transfusion, acute haemolytic reactions, circulatory overload, anaphylaxis and transfusion-related acute lung injury (TRALI). Bacterial or viral contamination can lead to recipient infection, eg hepatitis, and recurrent transfusion can lead to iron overload.

What would you say to a Jehovah's Witness who needs a blood transfusion?

If a patient has the capacity he or she is entitled to refuse any treatment, even if it would be life saving. Surgery can be performed using non-blood fluids, cell savers (recycling the patient's own blood) or blood substitutes (eg haemoglobin), but the patient should be made aware of the risks and benefits of surgery with and without the availability of blood transfusion. Other methods to promote the patient's own erythropoiesis (eg vitamin/iron supplements/erythropoietin) can be used.

What is meant by 'B symptoms'?

B symptoms are constitutional symptoms, properly only as part of the classification of lymphomas, but can also be considered in other diseases, eg with other cancers and autoimmune connective tissue diseases. They include fevers, night sweats and weight loss.

How would you classify CKD?

CKD is classified according to estimated glomerular filtration rate (eGFR), in addition to the presence/absence of glomerular haematuria/proteinuria and evidence of renal disease on imaging studies. The eGFR is calculated from the serum creatinine, and takes into account the patient's age, gender, and ethnicity:

Stage	eGFR	Other features
I	>90	(Only if abnormal imaging/proteinuria/haematuria)
II	60–90	(Only if abnormal imaging/proteinuria/haematuria)
III	30–59	IIIa – 45–59; IIIb – 30–44
IV	15–29	
V	<15	

If there is heavy proteinuria (urinary protein:creatinine >100 mg/mmol) then the letter 'P' can be added after the stage.

ENDOCRINE SYSTEM

DIABETES MELLITUS

Diabetes is becoming more common. Refer to type 1 and type 2 rather than insulin status – many patients with type 2 diabetes require insulin. Patients may be in hospital for treatment of diabetes or, more commonly, for treatment of its complications.

PC   Polydipsia/polyuria/thirst/weight loss
Coma (hypoglycaemia/DKA/HONK)
Eye disease (retinopathy/cataracts/retinal detachment)
Neuropathy
       Sensory polyneuropathy ('glove and stocking')
       Painful peripheral neuropathy (commonly leg pain)
       Autonomic neuropathy (impotence, gastroparesis with vomiting/diarrhoea, orthostatic symptoms)
       Mononeuropathy (eg mononeuritis multiplex)

HPC   When diagnosed/by whom/how?
Monitoring: blood sugar (BM)/urine dipstick
       How often? How good is control? Hypos?
Infections: UTI/*Candida* spp./ulcers/cellulitis

PMH   Hypertension/vascular disease (IHD/PVD/TIAs/CVA)
Kidney disease/eye disease

FH   Increased risk in relatives (type 2 > type 1)
At-risk ethnic groups (South Asian/Pacific Island/Black individuals)

SH   Smoking/diet

DH   Oral hypoglycaemic agents (metformin, sulphonylureas)
Insulin
       Type (human/porcine, long/short acting)
       Dose/timing (eg basal bolus regimen)
       Injection sites (? lipohypertrophy)

ROS Look specifically for any complications not already covered

EXAMINATION

General appearance

Well/unwell

Thin/obese

Fingerpricks from BM testing

CVS Blood pressure

Peripheral pulses (especially foot pulses)

Abdominal

Injection sites

CNS Visual acuity/fundoscopy (case 122)

Peripheral neuropathy (especially vibration sense/monofilament)

Absent ankle jerks/distal sensory loss

Peripheries

Necrobiosis lipoidica (case 85)

Ulcers: neuropathic/vascular

Diabetic foot: nail care, fungal infection, toe amputations

Urinalysis including specific testing for microalbuminuria

INVESTIGATIONS

In a patient presenting with complications the diagnosis is likely to have already been made. However, you should be aware of the WHO criteria (fasting blood glucose (FBG) >7.0 mmol/l or 2-h glucose >11.1 mmol/l; 2 h glucose >7.8 mmol/l is impaired glucose tolerance).

BM	**Rule out hypoglycaemia/DKA/HONK**
FBC/U&Es	Infection/dehydration/nephropathy
HbA1c	Measure of long-term BM control (about 3 months)
	Target <7.5% (<6.5% if CVS risk – most cases)
Cholesterol	For cardiovascular risk
C-peptide	To discriminate between type 1 and type 2
ABG	If DKA suspected

TREATMENT

For diabetic emergencies, see opposite

Patient education/CVS risk assessment (stop smoking)

Diet   All patients. There is no 'special' diabetic diet; more fresh fruit and vegetables, less saturated fat/salt/sugar

High BMs can be reduced by more drugs/less food

Oral hypoglycaemic agents (OHAs) for type 2 diabetes:

Metformin is first line (less weight gain/ fewer hypos)

Sulphonylureas added as second line

Gliptins/glitazones if sulphonylureas not tolerated/hypoglycaemia/if HbA1c remains >7.5%

Insulin for type 1 diabetes/in addition to OHAs in type 2

Long acting for background ('basal'), especially type 2

Short acting at mealtimes ('bolus'), especially type 1

Cholesterol: fibrates if hypertriglyceridaemia/statins

BP   Aim <135/85 mmHg if no albuminuria – use ACE inhibitors in type 2 diabetes

Aim <130/80 mmHg and use ACE inhibitors/ARBs if albuminuria

Primary prevention for CVS disease: aspirin 75 mg daily

Surveillance: at least annual eye and foot checks (type 1 diabetes)

EMERGENCIES

DKA/HONK

Precipitants: undertreatment (eg new diagnosis, infection)

Diagnosis: hyperglycaemia; ketonuria, acidosis (DKA)

Treatment: **rehydration** with 0.9% or physiological saline

Monitor and replace potassium **early**

DKA: **insulin** via intravenous infusion; **do not stop**

As BM drops (<15), add intravenous glucose

Hypoglycaemia

Oral high-sugar snack/drink if possible

If reduced consciousness, intravenous/intramuscular glucagon

If no improvement after 10 min, intravenous glucose

COMMENT

Diabetes mellitus is caused by a lack of insulin production (type 1) or insulin resistance (type 2):

Type 1   Younger patient/thin

Short history before diagnosis

Requires insulin

Remember that under physiological stress/illness insulin requirements **increase**, hence if patients continue/reduce their normal insulin they are at risk of DKA. They key feature is **lack of insulin** leading to tissue hypoglycaemia and ketone metabolism. Patients can be significantly dehydrated. Treatment is with **fluids** and **insulin**. Glucose is given to allow ongoing insulin therapy once the blood sugar has dropped.

Type 2   Middle-aged/overweight

Often 'subclinical' for some time before diagnosis – may present with complications

Treat with diet/weight loss/OHAs/insulin

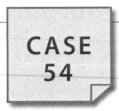

CASE 54

OBESITY AND THE METABOLIC SYNDROME

Obesity is becoming increasingly common across the western world. The metabolic syndrome (or syndrome X) may affect up to one in five people, and is increasingly screened for and diagnosed.

PC	May present desiring weight loss/due to complications
	May be identified by routine screening, eg health check
HPC	History of weight/blood pressure control
	Any complications: IHD/PVD/cerebrovascular/renal/hepatological/diabetes
PMH	Previous diagnosis of HTN/DM
FH	Type 2 diabetes/hypertension/dyslipidaemias
SH	Smoking
	Diet/exercise/alcohol consumption
DH	Antihypertensives/OHAs/lipid-lowering agents/primary prophylaxis with aspirin
	Drugs predisposing to weight gain, eg steroids

EXAMINATION

General appearance

Habitus – if possible measure weight and hip circumference

Weight and height – calculate BMI (weight in kg/(height in m)^2)

Jaundiced?

Rarely, may have acanthosis nigricans

? Underlying endocrine disorder (hypothyroid/Cushing's disease)

CVS

Blood pressure   Evidence of heart/vascular disease

Abdominal   Adiposity/striae

Urinalysis for glycosuria/microalbuminuria

INVESTIGATIONS

LFTs   Raised liver enzymes in fatty liver
Glucose (random/fasting/formal tolerance test)
Fasting lipid profile

TREATMENT

Conservative measures are paramount:

Dietary – more fresh fruit and vegetables, less salt, saturated fat, high-sugar foods and alcohol

Exercise – cardiovascular exercise sufficient to get out of breath for 30 min at least 3 days a week

Stop smoking

Medication for each individual component of the syndrome:

Antihypertensives (ACE inhibitors preferred if diabetic)

Lipid-lowering agents (statins for low HDL, fibrates for high triglycerides)

Metformin preferred if diabetic (less weight gain)

Treatment only if serious attempts at lifestyle modification have failed/been only partially successful:

Medical	Lipase inhibitors (reduce dietary fat absorption), eg orlistat
	Appetite suppressants, eg sibutramine
Surgical	Gastric banding/bypass

COMMENT

The following is the syndrome

Central obesity (waist >40 inches (102 cm) female/36 inches (91 cm) male or BMI > 30 kg/m²)

Plus two of

Hypertension

Dyslipidaemia (low serum HDL/raised triglycerides)

Raised fasting glucose (>5.6 mmol/l)/type 2 diabetes

± other features not required for diagnosis (microalbuminuria, non-alcoholic fatty liver disease, polycystic ovaries)

You should be aware of the concept of fat as an endocrine organ. Abnormal adipose tissue (eg hypertrophy in central obesity/loss in lipodystrophy) leads to insulin resistance and the metabolic syndrome. Exercise is beneficial for cardiovascular fitness and plasma lipids even if weight loss is not achieved.

HYPERTHYROIDISM/ GRAVES' DISEASE

A common disorder; although patients are often managed as outpatients, they frequently appear in finals examinations. About 25% of patients with Graves' thyroid disease develop eye disease.

PC   Extremely varied, often non-specific
        Palpitations/anxiety/tremor/heat intolerance
        Weight loss/GI upset/polydipsia/polyuria
        Weakness/fatigue/muscle aches/SOB

HPC   Symptoms may have been present for some time before diagnosis/investigated for other conditions
        Ask specifically about goitre/change in appearance

PMH   Autoimmune tendency

FH   Frequently history of thyroid/autoimmune disorders

DH   Treatment (β-blockers, carbimazole); cause (amiodarone)

ROS   Cover all the areas listed above

EXAMINATION

General appearance
        Thin/nervous/fidgety/dressed to keep cool

Hands Sweaty palms/palmar erythema/fine tremor
        Thyroid acropachy (case 72)

Neck   Goitre/? bruit

Face   Exophthalmos/lid retraction/lid lag/chemosis
        Often variable diplopia in Graves' disease (may mimic third nerve)
        Papilloedema/optic atrophy if prolonged

CVS	Tachycardia/bounding pulse/atrial fibrillation (case 7)
	Signs of heart failure (especially in elderly people)
CNS	Proximal muscle weakness (case 102)
Legs	Look for pretibial myxoedema (case 84)

INVESTIGATIONS

TFTs – high free T_4/T_3/low thyroid stimulating hormone

Thyroid antibodies – anti-TSH receptor in Graves' disease

Radioisotope studies – ? solitary nodule/general high uptake

TREATMENT

Block glandular T_4 synthesis – carbimazole

> Thyroid reserves of T_4 take some time to be exhausted
>
> Risk of agranulocytosis – warn patients to report infections; check FBC during initial treatment
>
> Can overblock – give T_4 ('block and replace')

Block peripheral T_3 conversion – propylthiouracil

β-blockers (propranolol) for symptomatic relief

Radioactive iodine – high efficacy, concentrates well in overactive gland, most become hypothyroid

Surgery if massive (airway obstructing) or cancerous gland: risk of laryngeal nerve palsy/hypoparathyroidism

COMMENT

'Thyroid storm' – acute, severe hyperthyroidism – is a medical emergency. Treatment is resuscitative with an ABCDE approach (see case 144), intravenous propranolol and steroids and radioactive iodine.

Causes   Graves' disease (stimulatory anti-TSH receptor antibodies)

Multinodular goitre (especially elderly people)

Solitary toxic nodule (Plummer's disease – about 5%)

De Quervain's thyroiditis – painful, tender thyroid with low radiolabelled iodine uptake; hyperthyroid period is followed by hypothyroidism before resolution. Treat symptoms and give NSAIDs

You need to distinguish those signs due to hyperthyroidism itself from those that occur only in Graves' disease (due to antibodies):

Graves' disease

Exophthalmos	Ocular muscle swelling
Pretibial myxoedema	'Waxy' swelling of shins
Thyroid acropachy	Resembles clubbing

HYPOTHYROIDISM

As with hyperthyroidism (case 55), symptoms can be vague and insidious. Note the patient's voice (hoarse/deepened).

PC   Dry skin/itch/decreased sweating/cold intolerance
Weight gain/fluid retention/constipation
Weakness/fatigue/muscle cramps/joint aches
Menstrual irregularity/loss of libido

HPC   Symptoms may have been present for some time before diagnosis/investigated for other conditions
Ask specifically about goitre/change in appearance

PMH   Autoimmune tendency

FH   Frequently history of thyroid/autoimmune disorders

DH   Treatment for hyperthyroidism (carbimazole, radiolabelled iodine)
Amiodarone/lithium therapy

E X A M I N A T I O N

General appearance
Overweight/slowed, hoarse, deepened 'breaking' voice
Dressed for cold weather, even indoors/hypothermia

Hands Carpal tunnel syndrome (case 73)
Brittle nails and hair

Neck   Goitre/? bruit
Previous thyroid surgery

Face   Loss of outer third of eyebrows (notoriously unreliable!)
Coarse facial features/xanthelasma
Periorbital puffiness

CVS   Bradycardia

CNS   Hypotonia/proximal muscle weakness
Slow-relaxing tendon reflexes

INVESTIGATIONS

FBC   Anaemia (normocytic/macrocytic with low vitamin B_{12})

TFTs   Low free T_4/T_3
TSH high if thyroid cause/low if pituitary

Thyroid antibodies

Anti-thyroid peroxidase/thyroglobulin in Hashimoto's thyroiditis

Pituitary function tests, eg prolactin

Cholesterol often raised (especially if xanthelasma)

TREATMENT

Thyroxine (T_4 replacement, should be levothyroxine): titrated to TFTs and symptoms

COMMENT

Causes

Hashimoto's thyroiditis – common (especially female)

Post-carbimazole/radiolabelled iodine/surgery

Pituitary disease (see case 60)

Iodine deficiency is the most common cause worldwide

Myxoedema coma is a rare presentation of severe hypothyroidism, especially in elderly people. Depressed consciousness, hypothermia, hypoventilation, cardiac failure and hypoglycaemia are common. Treatment is rescuscitative (ABCDE approach – see case 144) with intravenous T_3, steroids and glucose, and gradual rewarming.

The sick euthyroid syndrome frequently occurs in acute (and chronic) illness, eg infection, trauma, surgery, CKD, CCF. Thyroid hormone levels are low, but TSH is normal/low, and the patient is not clinically hypothyroid. It does not require treatment.

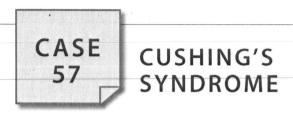

CASE 57
CUSHING'S SYNDROME

Introduce and expose

Observe   Habitus
Signs of any condition requiring steroids (eg SLE)

Face   Moon face/acne/hirsutism
Plethora
Oral candidiasis

Neck   Buffalo hump

Abdomen
Striae
Truncal ('centripetal') obesity

Peripheries
Limb muscle wasting
Thin skin with easy bruising

Extras   Urinalysis for glycosuria
Tell the examiner that you would like to take a history of steroid use

Causes	Iatrogenic	Most often prednisolone
	↑ ACTH	Pituitary microadenoma
		Ectopic (small-cell lung tumour (case 25))
	↓ ACTH	Adrenal tumour

COMMENT

Remember that Cushing's disease is only one cause of Cushing's syndrome, ie a pituitary ACTH-secreting adenoma. By far the most common cause of Cushing's syndrome is long-term steroid administration (iatrogenic Cushing's syndrome). Ensure that you look for signs of the underlying disease:

RA	Rheumatoid hands/nodules (case 63)
SLE	Malar 'butterfly' rash (case 64)
Chronic asthma	May have no signs/wheezy (case 22)
Pulmonary fibrosis	
	Fixed fine end-inspiratory crackles (case 23)
Transplantation	Scar of surgery (case 43)

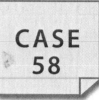

CASE 58

ADDISON'S DISEASE

As there are few clinical signs you may be given a clue in the history, eg the patient presents with malaise/weight loss/dizziness/abdominal pain.

Introduce and expose

Observe Female > male, young to middle-aged
Thin/tanned
Associated autoimmune disease – vitiligo, alopecia

Hands Pigmented skin creases (look at the palms)

Face Pigmented oral mucosa

CVS Postural hypotension
Tachycardia

INVESTIGATIONS

Cortisol   Low early morning cortisol may give a clue but is non-diagnostic

Short synacthen test (failure of adrenals to respond to ACTH) is more reliable

TREATMENT

Glucocorticoid replacement with prednisolone/hydrocortisone (shorter half-life, asymmetrically dosed to mimic diurnal variation of natural cortisol levels)
Mineralocorticoid replacement with fludrocortisone
Increased steroids needed when under physiological stress

COMMENT

Addison's disease as initially described was adrenal failure due to tuberculosis, but addisonism now refers to any cause of adrenal insufficiency. The most common cause is autoimmune – so look for associated autoimmune conditions such as type 1 diabetes and thyroid disease.

An addisonian crisis can occur after abrupt steroid withdrawal/new Addison's diagnosis/intercurrent illness without dose increase. Treatment is resuscitative (ABCDE approach – see case 144) with saline rehydration and intravenous hydrocortisone.

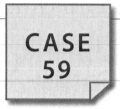

ACROMEGALY

If you are allowed to ask any questions, enquire about poorly fitting shoes/rings/gloves/hats.

Introduce and expose

Observe

Hands	Large 'spade-like' hands/no or tight rings Coarse skin Carpal tunnel syndrome (case 73)
Face	Broad nose/large ears/prominent supraorbital ridge Large jaw with mandibular prognathism (underbite) Interdental separation/large tongue
CNS	Bitemporal hemianopia (pituitary macroadenoma)
Extras	Urinalysis for glycosuria (associated diabetes)

INVESTIGATIONS

Growth hormone (GH) levels alone are unhelpful due to pulsatile secretion – blood levels vary from high to low even in normality.

GH – after glucose tolerance test (should suppress)
IGF-1 (insulin-like growth factor-1)
Other pituitary function tests – TSH, ACTH, prolactin
MRI of the brain (CT poorly sensitive due to base of skull)

TREATMENT

Medical treatment with somatostatin analogues (eg octreotide) or dopamine agonist (eg bromocriptine) can reduce GH levels and tumour size
Surgical removal (usually trans-sphenoidal)

COMMENT

GH-secreting tumours are usually macroadenomas, unlike ACTH-secreting tumours (compare with Cushing's disease).

Complications include diabetes, hypertension, heart disease and kidney disease (due to the GH excess), and visual field defects (bitemporal hemianopia from compression at the optic chiasma by tumour).

PANHYPO-PITUITARISM

Multiple pituitary deficiencies can result from tumour, compression, vascular insult or surgery/irradiation. Minor deficiencies may go unnoticed by the patient and clinician.

Symptoms and signs

Classically, 'alabaster skin' – pallor and hairlessness

Secondary hypothyroidism (case 56)

Secondary hypoadrenalism (case 58)

Secondary hypogonadism – loss of libido, secondary sexual hair, amenorrhoea, impotence

Few symptoms/signs from GH/prolactin deficiency

Posterior pituitary – ADH deficiency (diabetes insipidus) may be masked by coexistent hypoadrenalism

Non-specific symptoms can predominate

Visual field defects (bitemporal hemianopia) suggest tumour

Causes

Malignancy – primary/secondary

Trauma – especially surgery

Fibrosis – post-radiotherapy

Infection – meningitis/encephalitis

Infarction/haemorrhage – 'pituitary apoplexy'

Infiltration – sarcoidosis, haemochromatosis

INVESTIGATIONS

Endocrine function tests – TFTs, sex steroids, LH, FSH, ACTH and cortisol, IGF-1/GH-stimulation test

MRI of the brain

TREATMENT

Replace steroids and thyroid hormone urgently
Sex steroid replacement ± gonadotrophins for fertility
GH replacement improves quality of life and muscle mass
DDAVP (desmopressin) intranasally for diabetes insipidus

COMMENT

Pituitary apoplexy is sudden, dramatic panhypopituitarism caused by pituitary infarction/haemorrhage (vascular accident/into tumour).

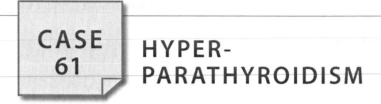

CASE 61
HYPER-PARATHYROIDISM

This is generally a biochemical diagnosis with few clinical signs or symptoms. Hyperparathyroidism (hyperPTH) can be primary, secondary or tertiary.

Symptoms of hypercalcaemia
'Stones, bones, abdominal moans and psychic groans'
> Renal stones: loin pain
> Bone/muscle pain/osteoporosis
> Polydipsia/polyuria
> Anorexia/constipation/nausea and vomiting
> Weakness/fatigue/depression
> Cognitive impairment

Signs of CKD (case 42)
> Suggest secondary/tertiary hyperPTH

Urinalysis
> For microscopic haematuria with renal stones

INVESTIGATIONS

> U&Es   Renal failure with dehydration/CKD as cause
> LFTs   ALP may be elevated (increased bone turnover in secondary)
> Calcium level elevated (primary/tertiary)
> Phosphate level decreased (primary)/elevated (secondary/tertiary)
> PTH

TREATMENT

Treat hypercalcaemia: saline diuresis/bisphosphonates
PTH suppression with vitamin D analogues (secondary/tertiary)
Calcimimetics (secondary/tertiary)
Surgical parathyroidectomy for a single adenoma/failed medical treatment for secondary/tertiary – a complex operation, because the parathyroids may vary in number and position

SEQUELAE

Hypoparathyroidism; laryngeal nerve palsy

COMMENT

Primary hyperPTH is usually due to a single functional adenoma. Secondary hyperPTH occurs with chronic vitamin D deficiency, eg CKD, and is an appropriate response to low serum calcium. If left unchecked, the parathyroid becomes autonomous and fails to suppress even with normal Ca^{2+} – tertiary hyperPTH.

EXAMINATION OF THYROID STATUS

As treatment for hyperthyroidism can cause hypothyroidism, and vice versa, and some thyroid diseases can have periods of both (De Quervain's thyroiditis and acute Hashimoto's thyroiditis); often you will simply be asked to examine a patient's thyroid status. Follow a systematic routine.

Introduce and expose in such a way that the patient answers you. Listen for the hoarse/deepened 'breaking' voice of hypothyroidism.

	Hyperthyroid	**Hypothyroid**
Observe	Thin	Overweight
	Underdressed	Overdressed
	Fidgety/nervous	Slowed
Hands	Sweaty/red palms	Brittle nails
	Fine tremor	Carpal tunnel syndrome
Pulse	Tachycardia/AF	Bradycardia
Face	Lid lag/retraction	Loss of outer third of eyebrow
	Chemosis (injected eye)	Xanthelasma
		Puffy, coarse facies
Neck	Goitre ± bruit	Goitre ± bruit

Feel the neck from behind at rest, then ask the patient to take a sip of water and hold it in their mouth. Feel again as he or she swallows.

Peripheries

	Proximal weakness	Proximal weakness
		Slow-relaxing reflexes

Autoimmune thyroid disease is associated with other autoimmune conditions – look for vitiligo and alopecia. There are many other associated conditions (eg scleroderma, coeliac disease, pernicious anaemia, type 1 diabetes mellitus, Addison's disease).

VIVA QUESTIONS

What is meant by insulin resistance?

Failure of peripheral tissues to respond adequately to insulin, and hence hyperglycaemia, is described as insulin resistance. This is putatively due to poor responsiveness to insulin by abnormal peripheral fat cells, eg in obesity, older age or lipodystrophy. Treatments are aimed at increasing insulin sensitivity with lifestyle changes (eg weight loss, exercise) or drugs (eg metformin).

Tell me about hypoglycaemia in type 1 diabetes

In type 1 diabetes mellitus there is an absolute lack of insulin due to the destruction of the β cells of the pancreatic islets. The patient requires supplementary insulin to utilise glucose and prevent ketoacidosis. However, if the dose of insulin is too high relative to the blood sugar, hypoglycaemia can develop. Generally patients are aware when they are becoming 'hypo', developing adrenergic symptoms such as sweating, shaking, palpitations and paraesthesiae. Patients should have a high-sugar drink or snack available to rapidly increase plasma glucose and overcome the symptoms, then consider longer-acting carbohydrates and a review of insulin dose to prevent attacks.

Patients with frequent 'hypos' may develop hypoglycaemia unawareness, which can be life threatening because they are unable to identify and respond to hypoglycaemic episodes early.

Describe the use of insulin

Insulin is given subcutaneously in the maintenance treatment of diabetes, or intravenously for diabetic comas or as part of a 'sliding scale' to continually deliver insulin in a fasted patient, eg pre-theatre. Short-, medium- and long-acting insulins are available, and patients should have access to their own formulations of insulin to prevent too great a variability in their blood sugars. Insulin is also used in the management of acute hyperkalaemia.

Insulin's immediate effects are increasing the uptake of glucose, amino acids and potassium into insulin-sensitive cells. Medium-term effects include protein synthesis/inhibition of degradation, increased glucagon synthesis and decreased hepatic gluconeogenesis. Long-term effects include increasing expression of mRNA for lipogenic enzymes.

Is hypercalcaemia a cause or consequence of dehydration?

Both. Hypercalcaemia can lead to a natriuresis, and hence dehydration, but the kidney also requires a good tubular flow to excrete calcium well. Treatment for hypercalcaemia of any cause therefore includes saline diuresis to rehydrate the patient and maximise renal calcium excretion.

What is Addison's disease?

The disease as first described by Addison was adrenal failure as a consequence of tuberculous infection. Most commonly now it is due to autoimmune destruction of the glands, or iatrogenic addisonism after abrupt withdrawal of exogenous corticosteroids. The lack of mineralocorticoid activity leads to salt and water wasting in the distal tubule, with retention of potassium. Lack of glucocorticoid activity can lead to hypoglycaemia, and dehydration can lead to hypercalcaemia. Treatment is with replacement of steroids (hydrocortisone) and salt and water (physiological saline).

How would you recognise a patient with acromegaly? What questions would you ask?

Growth hormone stimulates skeletal and soft-tissue growth. This causes gigantism in children (if it develops before epiphyseal fusion) and acromegaly in adults (usually due to a pituitary adenoma). The patient will have a prominent supraorbital ridge, large nose/bridge and a protruding lower jaw with malocclusion and interdental separation of the teeth. There may be macroglossia, large 'spade-like' hands and feet with spatulate digits. More formal examination may reveal a bitemporal hemianopia, hidrosis, greasy skin, cardiomegaly and goitre.

One can enquire about changes in facial appearance; shoe, glove and hat size; rings that no longer fit; headaches and visual deterioration; or complications (eg diabetes, cardiac failure).

What diagnoses would you consider in a patient with persistent generalised lymphadenopathy: (1) in a 25-year-old and (2) in a 65-year-old?

The causes of generalised lymphadenopathy are haematological (lymphoma, chronic lymphocytic leukaemia (CLL), acute leukaemia), infective (EBV, HIV, toxoplasmosis, TB, brucellosis, secondary syphilis) or other (SLE, rheumatoid, sarcoid and drugs, eg phenytoin).

A 25-year-old and 65-year-old may both have lymphoma (with Hodgkin's lymphoma more common in young and diffuse large B-cell non-Hodgkin's lymphoma in elderly people), but the former is more likely to have EBV, HIV or, given the resurgence, syphilis. CLL is a disorder of the over-50s and acute leukaemias are statistically more common in this age group.

THE MUSCULOSKELETAL SYSTEM

Examination of the musculoskeletal system

'Examine this patient's hands'

There are many diagnoses that may be picked up when examining a patient's hands. Develop a systematic routine so as not to miss any.

Introduce and expose
Try to have the hands and forearms fully visible, relaxed in the patient's lap/on a pillow

Observe Cachexia

Psoriatic rash (elbows/extensor surfaces/scalp)

Face	Cushingoid (case 57)	Steroid use, eg RA, SLE
	Exophthalmos	Thyroid acropachy (Graves' disease, case 55)
	Acromegaly (case 59)	Carpal tunnel syndrome/nerve thickening/diabetic neuropathy
	Heliotrope rash	Dermatomyositis
	Microstomia	Systemic sclerosis (case 68)
	Telangiectasis	Systemic sclerosis
	Red eyes	Uveitis/scleritis/episcleritis

Hands

Nails	Clubbing (case 72)	Could also be thyroid acropachy
	Splinters	Endocarditis (case 6)
	Leukonychia	Hypoalbuminaemia
	Nail bed infarcts	RA/systemic sclerosis
	Pitting/ridging	Psoriasis
Skin	Tight	Systemic sclerosis
	Steroidal	
	Raynaud's phenomenon	
	Spider naevi (case 36)	
	Gouty tophi (case 71)	

Rash of dermatomyositis (case 81)
Tendon xanthomas

Palms   Palmar pigmentation/erythema
Dupuytren's contracture

Joints   Observe   Swelling/inflammation/deformity
Palpate   Tenderness (metacarpal squeeze)/synovial
thickening/Heberden's or Osler's nodes

Nerves   Wasting   Interossei/thenar/hypothenar
Weakness   First dorsal interosseus (ulnar)/abductor
pollicis brevis (median)
Sensation   Pinprick/joint position/vibration
Differentiate ulnar/median/radial/C6, C7–C8

Function   Undo and do up buttons/write/hold a cup, etc

Wrists   Peripheral pulses
'Piano keying' (ulnar subluxation)

Elbows   Gouty tophi (case 71)
Rheumatoid nodules (case 63)
Psoriatic plaques (case 77)
Tendon xanthomas

Neck   Restricted movement/'question mark' posture (case 69)

Back   Kyphosis/scoliosis
Loss of height   Vertebral collapse (osteoporosis)
Reduced movement   Ankylosing spondylitis (case 69)

Legs   Bowed   Paget's disease (case 70)
Previous hip/knee surgery (osteoarthritis (case 66)/
osteoporotic fracture (case 67))

Feet   Pes cavus
Toenail clubbing

RHEUMATOID ARTHRITIS

Remember that the inflammatory arthritides are characterised by pain worse after rest and relieved by use. The patient may be admitted due to the joint disease, extra-articular disease or complications of treatment.

PC **Joint pain/swelling/stiffness**
Fatigue/malaise

HPC Which joints are affected (**symmetrical** pattern)?
'Early morning stiffness' – duration?
Acute swelling/effusion
Extra-articular complications:

Chest pain	Pericarditis
SOB	Pleural effusion/pulmonary fibrosis/anaemia
Dry/red eye	Sjögren's syndrome/scleritis
Neurological	Nerve entrapment/Carpal tunnel syndrome/peripheral neuropathy
Skin	Nodules/Raynaud's phenomenon/ulceration

PMH GORD/peptic ulceration/CKD (care with NSAIDs)

FH Familial in 5–10%

SH **Functional ability** for activities of daily living – buttons/self-care
Any aids at home/for mobility/wheelchair use

DH Treatments past and present
Response to previous treatment? Side-effects?
Ask about joint injections/depot injections (steroids)

ROS Constitutional symptoms

EXAMINATION

General appearance

Female (three times more common than in men)
Pale/tired/unwell/febrile
Lymphadenopathy

Hands   All joints must be examined for:

Swelling	Synovitis/effusion
Pain	Remember metacarpal squeeze
Erythema	
Limitation of movement/function	
Deformity	Swan-neck/boutonnière/Z-deformity of thumb/ulnar deviation of fingers

Rheumatoid nodules over extensor tendons (RhF positive)

Face   Dry/red eyes/scleritis/scleromalacia

CVS   Pericardial rub (case 4)

Respiratory

Pleural effusion (case 27)/Fibrosis (case 23 – from disease/treatments)

Abdomen

Splenomegaly (case 46 – Felty's syndrome)

CNS   Carpal tunnel syndrome (case 73)/peripheral neuropathy (case 103)

Legs   Pyoderma gangrenosum (case 83)/erythema nodosum (case 82)

Look at the knees and feet

Urinalysis for proteinuria (drugs/amyloid)

INVESTIGATIONS

FBC   Anaemia (chronic disease/blood loss secondary NSAIDs)

U&Es   Renal impairment secondary to many disease-modifying anti-rheumatic drugs (DMARDs)/NSAIDs

CRP   Marker of disease activity

RhF   For diagnosis; ANAs may also be present
Anti-cyclic citrullinated peptide (CCP) antibodies if clinical
suspicion but RhF negative
Joint aspiration if suspicion of septic arthritis
Hands/feet radiograph if persistent synovitis of small joints

RADIOLOGICAL FINDINGS

Soft-tissue swelling/loss of joint space
Periarticular osteopenia/erosions
Subluxation/frank deformity

TREATMENT

Treatment should ideally be initiated with 3 months of
developing persistent symptoms to reduce progression
Multidisciplinary approach with physiotherapy, podiatry, etc
Combination therapy with:

Glucocorticoids – for new diagnosis/flares
Methotrexate
One other DMARD, eg sulfasalazine,
hydroxychloroquine, gold, penicillamine

If treatment failure on these, TNF-α inhibitors (eg infliximab) or
other biologic agents (eg rituximab)
Intra-articular steroids for large joints
Symptom control with:

NSAIDs for short courses/low doses + PPI cover
Paracetamol/codeine preparations

Surgical referral if persistent/unmanageable symptoms or
specific indication, eg carpal tunnel syndrome

COMMENT

Contrast rheumatoid arthritis with osteoarthritis (case 66)

	Rheumatoid arthritis	**Osteoarthritis**
Morning stiffness	Common, usually >1 h	Rarer, usually <1 h
Joint involvement	PIP/MCP joints of hands	DIP joints of hands
	Large joints less common	Spine, hips, knees but any can be affected
Blood tests	Inflammatory markers	None specific

Side-effects of anti-rheumatic drugs:

Steroids	Weight gain/Cushing's syndrome/thin skin/bruising/osteoporosis/peptic ulcer disease
Joint injection	Infection/ulceration
DMARDs	Myelosuppression – monitor FBC, educate patient to attend if any signs of infection
	Proteinuria/interstitial nephritis – monitor
	Hepatic/pulmonary fibrosis (methotrexate)
	Visual impairment (hydroxychloroquine)
	Many others (eg GI upset, headache)
TNF-α inhibitors	Infections (including TB)/hypersensitivity
Rituximab	Infusion reactions
NSAIDs	Peptic ulceration/interstitial nephritis

SYSTEMIC LUPUS ERYTHEMATOSUS

Patients are usually young females, and tend to be well informed about their condition – use their expertise.

PC   Often **arthralgia/rash,** but see below

HPC   Initial diagnosis: when/precipitating event?
SLE is extremely variable in its manifestation, and a truly multisystem disorder. Your systemic enquiry will be exhausted during this part of the history.

General Fever/malaise/fatigue

CVS   Peri-/myo-/endocarditis/early atheroma/IHD

Respiratory
             Pleural effusions/pleurisy/interstitial lung disease

GI   Anorexia/weight loss/mouth ulcers

GU   Nephrotic syndrome/CKD

Musculoskeletal
             Arthralgia/myalgia/(usually non-deforming) arthritis

Neurological
             Headache/stroke/seizures/mononeuropathy

Psychological
             Depression/psychosis/acute confusional states

Skin   Malar 'butterfly' rash/photosensitivity/discoid lupus/hair loss

PMH   Recurrent miscarriages/DVT/PE

FH   Ethnicity: Black > Asian > White
             Familial tendency (though not a simple single gene disorder)

DH   Drugs causing lupus-like syndromes (eg procainamide)

SH   Affects on lifestyle – ask specifically about sun avoidance

EXAMINATION

General appearance

Female (nine times more common than in men), usually young
Pallor/pyrexia/lymphadenopathy
Discoid lupus/vasculitic rash

Hands Raynaud's phenomenon
Nail-bed infarcts/finger spindling (scleroderma like)

Face Malar rash (sun sensitive)
Dry/gritty eyes (Sjögren's syndrome)

CVS Hypertension (related to renal disease)
Aseptic (Libman–Sacks syndrome) endocarditis – rare

Respiratory

Pleural rub/effusion

Musculoskeletal

Often normal (despite severe pain)/non-deformed
Acute joint swelling
A few patients have rheumatoid-like hand/foot deformity

CNS Mononeuritis multiplex
Signs of previous CVA (thrombotic tendency)

Urinalysis for proteinuria/haematuria as sign of lupus nephritis

INVESTIGATIONS

FBC Anaemia of chronic disease/leukopenia/
thrombocytopenia

U&Es Renal disease

ESR Elevated (marker of disease activity)

CRP Often normal (raised may indicate added infection)

Coagulation
APTT elevated ('lupus anticoagulant' –
thrombosis)

ANA 99% sensitive but only 50% specific (absence rules out)
Anti-dsDNA 70% sensitive but 95% specific (diagnostic)
Other autoantibodies (RhF, anti-Sm, anti-Ro, anti-La)

Anti-phospholipid/Anti-cardiolipin antibodies (thrombosis)
Complement components (C3/C4) low in active disease
False-positive VDRL (syphilis serology)
ECG/chest radiograph
Laboratory urinalysis ± renal biopsy if abnormal dipstick

TREATMENT
Patient education
Sun avoidance/sunblock for photosensitivity
Glucocorticoids – for flares
Hydroxychloroquine as maintenance/steroid sparing
Lupus nephritis/cerebral vasculitis may require cyclophosphamide + anti-proliferative (eg azathioprine, mycophenolate)
Symptom control with:
> NSAIDs for pain (**avoid** if renal disease) + PPI cover
> Paracetamol/codeine preparations

Anti-phospholipid syndrome – warfarin for venous thrombosis/aspirin for arterial thrombosis

COMMENT

Lupus is a notorious mimic of other conditions (eg endocarditis, pleural effusion, stroke) – have a high index of suspicion and a low threshold for testing ANAs.

There is a distinct overlap between the autoimmune connective tissue diseases, and this often confuses candidates and examiners alike. Mixed connective tissue disease (MCTD) is a useful term in cases where there are features of more than one of: SLE, systemic sclerosis (case 68), rheumatoid arthritis (case 63) and polymyositis (case 81). The ANA pattern is typically speckled, with the specific antibodies against the extractable nuclear anti-ribonucleoprotein antigen (anti-RNP).

Sjögren's syndrome is commonly associated with SLE/RA/scleroderma, although it can exist as a disease in its own right. The predominant symptoms are mucosal dryness (sicca syndrome) – dry, gritty, red eyes and dry mouth (xerostomia).

MULTIPLE MYELOMA

The varied nature of the symptoms means that the patient may present to a variety of specialists, eg orthopaedic surgeons, general physicians, haematologists and nephrologists.

PC	Bone pain/pathological fracture
	Malaise/fatigue/constitutional symptoms
	Infection (presenting symptom in about 10%) – pneumonia, UTI
HPC	Pain in back/ribs; worse with activity
	Tenderness/continuous well-localised pain (? fracture)
	Symptoms of hypercalcaemia (especially GI/neuropsychiatric)
	Time course – often chronic/insidious/worsening
PMH	May be preceded by monoclonal gammopathy of unknown significance (MGUS) (blood tests monitored for 'abnormal blood protein' before diagnosis)

EXAMINATION

General appearance

Usually older patient

Easy bruising

Pale/tired/unwell

In pain on movement (secondary to pathological fracture)

Dehydrated (especially hypercalcaemia)/uraemic

CVS   Rarely, heart failure secondary to hyperviscosity

Respiratory

? Pneumonia (case 24)

Abdominal

Hepatomegaly/splenomegaly/both (amyloid)

Musculoskeletal
Examine the back:
Erythema ab igne (case 86) – chronic pain
Vertebral collapse with loss of height/kyphosis
Peripheral oedema (nephrotic syndrome – amyloid)

CNS   Peripheral neuropathy/cord compression may occur
Urinalysis for proteinuria/haematuria/UTI

INVESTIGATIONS
FBC   Normochromic/normocytic anaemia/low platelets
U&Es   Renal impairment
LFTs, albumin and total protein, calcium
ESR   Raised
Immunoglobulins and electrophoresis for M-band:
Quantification and identification of any
paraprotein
Urinalysis for Bence Jones protein
Radiographs – skeletal survey
Bone marrow biopsy for clonal plasma cell infiltrates

TREATMENT
Pain relief with paracetamol/opioids – try to avoid NSAIDs
Rehydration (hypercalcaemia/renal failure)
Treat infections aggressively (broad-spectrum antibiotics)
Specific treatment depends on co-morbidity/frailty:
Melphalan + prednisolone
Cyclophosphamide + dexamethasone
Thalidomide may be added
Bortezimib (Velcade)

COMMENT

Monoclonal gammopathy of unknown significance (MGUS) is common and increases with age, occurring in 5% of those aged >80. The monoclonal protein (M-protein) may be whole immunoglobulin or light chains only. About 1% per year will progress to myeloma.

Suspect a myeloma/other plasma cell disorder (plasmacytoma/ Waldenström's macroglobulinaemia) if there is a raised ESR/anaemia or other signs of myelosuppression/low immunoglobulins (immunoparesis)/ unexplained renal failure/hypercalcaemia.

MGUS	Asymptomatic – myeloma	Symptomatic
M-protein <30 g/l	M-protein >30 g/l	Any M-protein
<10% plasma cells	>10% plasma cells	Any plasma cells
No organ damage	No organ damage	Any organ damage
No amyloid		

Organ damage may be bone/hypercalcaemia/bone marrow/renal or a tendency to infection (more than two bacterial infections in 12 months).

OSTEOARTHRITIS

The signs in the hands are most helpful. Although joints can be stiff, pain worsens over the course of the day/with use (compare rheumatoid arthritis – case 63).

Introduce and expose

Observe   Usually middle-aged, female

Hands   Heberden's nodes (bony swelling of DIPs)
Bouchard's nodes (bony swelling of PIPs)
Squaring of hands (first carpometacarpal joint)
Surgical scars

Nerves

Function may be decreased

Other joints for crepitus/scars of joint replacement/swelling

RADIOLOGICAL FINDINGS

Osteophytes and 'spurs'
Subchondral cysts/sclerosis

TREATMENT

Graded exercise (physiotherapy referral)
Weight loss if overweight
Analgesics – paracetamol as first line, NSAIDs in need
? Glucosamine sulphate (selected patients only)

Causes

Primary   Middle-aged women/familial/predominant DIP joint involvement

Secondary

Any cause of joint damage:

Wear and tear	Obesity/manual labour/runners, etc
Disabled patients	In arm of crutch use
Inflammatory arthritides (RA/gout/others)	
Neuropathic (Charcot's) joints, eg diabetes	

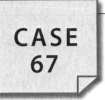

CASE 67 OSTEOPOROSIS

Symptoms

Often none

Back pain/radicular pain

Loss of height

Introduce and expose

Observe Commonly postmenopausal woman

More common in White/Asian people

Signs of long-term steroid therapy

Back **Loss of height**/kyphosis/scoliosis

Rib fractures

Extras Wrist/hip 'fragility' fractures

Risk factors

Familial tendency

Increasing age (especially after the menopause)

Oestrogen/testosterone deficiency (eg premature ovarian failure/hypogonadotrophic hypogonadism)

Glucocorticoid use

Hyperparathyroidism (case 61)

Malnutrition/vitamin D deficiency

Inactivity/low body mass

Low peak bone mass, eg low activity levels in youth

INVESTIGATIONS

Dual x-ray absorptiometry (DXA) scanning to calculate T-score (number of standard deviations below mean bone density):

$T < -2.5$	Osteoporosis
$T -2.5$ to -1	Osteopenia

TREATMENT

Weight-bearing exercise
Adequate diet
Calcium/vitamin D supplementation
Bisphosphonates

SYSTEMIC SCLEROSIS

The disease can be limited (cutaneous) or diffuse (systemic). The peripheral signs of scleroderma are paramount.

Introduce and expose

Observe Signs of mixed connective tissue disease (case 64)
Wearing gloves indoors?

Hands Tight/shiny/'spindle-shaped' fingers
Raynaud's phenomenon
Calcinosis
Finger pulp/nail-bed infarcts
Ulcers/autoamputation
Joint swelling
Carpal tunnel syndrome/proximal muscle weakness

Face 'Hooked' nose
Tight skin around mouth/'pursed lips' (microstomia)
Telangiectasia

Chest Pulmonary fibrosis (case 23)/hypertension

Extras Examine the other joints

COMMENT

Systemic sclerosis is a multisystem disease that can affect the GI tract, cardiorespiratory system and kidneys, in addition to the skin and joints. Organ dysfunction is the major cause of mortality.

Remember the CREST syndrome:

Calcinosis

Raynaud's phenomenon

Oesophageal reflux/stricture

Scleroderma

Telangiectasia

Raynaud's phenomenon often shows cyclical 'red, white and blue' changes in the fingers – hypoperfusion due to vascular spasm (white), becoming cyanosed when severe (blue), then hyperaemic with paraesthesia when reperfused (red). Treatment is with cold avoidance (eg gloves), vasodilator antihypertensives (eg nifedipine) and in severe cases sympathectomy.

ANKYLOSING SPONDYLITIS

There may be a hint in the examiner's instruction – unlike most other joint diseases, ankylosing spondylitis predominantly affects the axial skeleton. You might be asked to examine the neck/back, or to watch the patient walk/look at the ceiling.

Introduce and expose

Observe	Usually young/middle-aged
	Male (three times more common than in women)
Posture	'Question mark' posture: loss of lumbar lordosis, kyphosis and extension of the cervical spine
	Protuberant abdomen
Neck	Rigid spine – unable to turn head without turning whole body/ unable to touch shoulder with ear
Back	Reduced movement, eg on bending forward
	Unable to stand straight against a wall (ie with heels, buttocks, shoulder blades and occiput against the wall)

Associated features – say you would like to examine for the '5 As':

Anterior uveitis
Apical lung fibrosis
Aortic regurgitation/aortitis
Achilles tendinitis/plantar fasciitis
Arthritis – usually oligoarthritis of the large joints (eg knee)

INVESTIGATIONS

Radiographs may show spondylitis/'bamboo spine'

TREATMENT

Physiotherapy and mobility exercises are the mainstay

Analgesics

Anti-rheumatics

COMMENT

Spondyloarthropathy can also occur with psoriasis (case 77), inflammatory bowel disease (case 37) and Reiter's syndrome (reactive arthritis). Almost all patients are HLA-B27 positive.

PAGET'S DISEASE

You may be asked to examine the patient's face or legs. The symptoms are caused by dysregulated bone turnover and growth.

Face

Introduce and expose

Observe Increased size of skull
Hearing aid
There may be other cranial nerve lesions due to compression as they leave the many skull foramina:
Poor vision/optic atrophy (angioid streaks)
Sixth nerve palsy

Legs

Introduce and expose

Observe Bowing of the tibia (anteriorly – usually unilateral)

Palpate Warmth (high blood flow)

Auscultate Bruit

Symptoms Bone pain/headache/fatigue

INVESTIGATIONS

ALP Elevated with normal calcium/phosphate/PTH

COMMENT

Sir James Paget described a number of diseases; this is most properly called Paget's disease of bone. The differential diagnosis is of syphilitic sabre tibia and rickets. Rickets is usually bilateral and syphilis is rare.

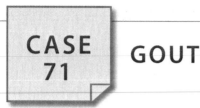

CASE 71 GOUT

Introduce and expose

Observe Obesity (BMI >35 kg/m^2 gives a three times risk of gout)
Ruddy 'boozer's' face

Hands **Tophi** (yellow/white subcutaneous nodules over joints)
Skin thinned/ulcerated over tophi
Asymmetrical swelling of the small joints
May be acutely inflamed/tender

Elbows Tophi

Face Tophi on ear

Feet Similar picture to the hands
The hallux is most often affected in acute gout

INVESTIGATIONS

Uric acid levels raised (although this is not sensitive/specific)
U&Es   Renal failure as a cause/consequence
Joint aspiration for an acutely swollen, hot, tender joint:
Needle-shaped negatively birefringent urate crystals
Rule out septic arthritis

TREATMENT

Diet and lifestyle advice (lose weight, reduce alcohol intake)

Withdraw any exacerbating drugs (eg thiazide diuretics)

For an acute flare: anti-inflammatories:

NSAIDs can be very effective

Colchicine (limited by development of diarrhoea)

Short course of steroids if unsuccessful

For prophylaxis **after** a flare has settled:

Allopurinol

COMMENT

Occasionally there is gross deformity of the joints due to tophus formation and joint margin erosions.

Differential diagnosis of lumps on the elbow: rheumatoid nodules.

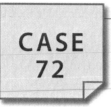

CASE 72 CLUBBING

Introduce and expose

Observe Signs of underlying disease

Hands **Loss of angle** of the nail bed ('diamond sign' negative)
Increased AP and lateral curvature of the nail
Fluctuation of the nail-bed/soft-tissue 'drumsticking'

Feet Look for clubbing of the toes

Look carefully for any clues to an underlying cause.

Causes

Idiopathic	Most common	No signs
Lung	Suppurative lung disease	Sputum (bronchiectasis) Cystic fibrosis (case 26) Fever (abscess/empyema)
	Pulmonary fibrosis (case 23)	Dyspnoea; fixed fine end- expiratory crackles
	Bronchial carcinoma	Tar staining/cachexia
Heart	Cyanotic congenital heart disease (case 16)	Down's syndrome; cardiac surgery scar
	Endocarditis (case 6) Atrial myxoma	Splinter haemorrhages
Abdominal	Cirrhosis	Signs of liver disease (case 36)
	Crohn's disease/colitis (case 37) Coeliac disease	Malnourished
Endocrine	Thyroid acropachy	Graves' disease (case 55)

Remember hypertrophic pulmonary osteoarthropathy can resemble clubbing – tenderness on squeezing wrists/other joints, may have enlargement of the extremities/coarse skin, association with bronchial carcinomas (case 25).

UPPER LIMB NERVE LESIONS

Ulnar/median nerve/T1 root lesions often appear as an 'Examine this patient's hands' case in finals.

Introduce and expose	Ulnar	Median	**T1**
Observe	Clawing fourth and fifth fingers		
Wasting	Hypothenar, interossei	Thenar	All small muscles
Weakness	Ad-/Abduction of fingers	Abductor pollicis brevis	All small muscles
Sensory loss	Fifth/medial half of fourth finger	Lateral 3½ fingers	Medial forearm
Extras	Deformed elbow rheumatoid	Tinel's sign over carpal tunnel; scar at wrist	Lymph nodes; ipsilateral Horner's syndrome

Median/ulnar nerves may be damaged anywhere along their course (compression/trauma) or be affected by a mononeuropathy. Common causes are carpal tunnel syndrome (median) and compression at the elbow, eg RA/crutch use (median/ulnar).

T1 root lesions may be due to damage at the:

Cord (especially bilateral)	Syringomyelia (case 100)/tumour
Root	Cervical spondylosis
Brachial plexus	Pancoast (apical lung) tumour

(associated with Horner's syndrome (case 112)/cachexia, etc)

Radial nerve lesions are less common. The clinical features are sensory loss over the anatomical snuffbox (lateral dorsum of the hand) and adjacent forearm, and motor weakness of the extensors of the wrist and fingers giving wrist drop ('Saturday night palsy').

NECK

Examination of the neck

'Examine this patient's neck' usually indicates one of four possibilities:

1. Abnormal JVP
2. Cervical lymphadenopathy
3. Goitre ± abnormal thyroid status (case 62)
4. Ankylosing spondylitis (case 69)

If the patient is seated on a chair that you can get behind and/or there is a glass of water nearby, it is most likely to be a goitre and least likely to be an abnormal JVP. If the patient is on a bed at 45° or able to lean back then the opposite is true. This is a difficult case. However, if you are methodical you will not miss anything.

Introduce and expose

Observe	Thyroid eye disease	Exophthalmos (Graves' disease)
		Lid lag/retraction
	Glass of water nearby	
	Dyspnoea/oedema	Cor pulmonale
	Wasting	Malignancy/lymphadenopathy
Inspect	Obvious goitre?	Go to case 74
	JVP	Go to case 76
	'Question mark' posture of ankylosing spondylitis	
Palpate	Midline swelling	Thyroglossal cyst – ask the patient to stick out the tongue while you palpate; a cyst will move upwards
		Otherwise go to case 74
	Palpable nodes	Go to case 75

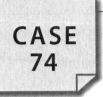

CASE 74 — GOITRE

Palpate the mass from behind

    ? Single nodule/multinodular/diffusely enlarged

    Any associated lymphadenopathy?

Ask the patient to take a sip of water and hold it in their mouth

Palpate again as they swallow

    A goitre should move up

Percuss down to the sternum (retrosternal goitre)

Auscultate for a bruit

If time allows, examine the thyroid status (case 62)/state that you would like to do so

Similarly, look for eye signs (case 120)/state that you would like to

COMMENT

To fully revise the thyroid look at cases 55, 56, 62 and 120.

CASE 75

LYMPH-ADENOPATHY

Ask the patient to sit forwards.

Palpate each of the neck areas in turn **from behind**

    Superior and deep cervical chains

    Horizontal ring

    Supraclavicular fossae

Describe any lump/bumps as you would any 'surgical' mass:

    Site/size/shape/surface

    Temperature/tethering/tenderness

    Contour/colour/consistency, etc

State that you would like to examine the other lymph node areas (axillary/inguinal).

The most common diagnoses are:

Reactive node(s)	Recent upper respiratory tract infection/fever
Neoplasia/metastases	Cachexia
Lymphoma	B symptoms
Tuberculosis	

It is almost impossible to describe in print the difficult job of assessing the JVP. We strongly advise you to arrange bedside teaching before the exam, which is by far the best way to understand what is going on. Many inpatient specialities (cardiology, respiratory, renal) will have patients with abnormal JVP.

Lean the patient back at 45°.

Observe Is the JVP visible? (Right side of neck is easiest)

Measure the height in centimetres above the sternal angle

Time pulsation against the opposite carotid pulse

If not visible:

Is it above the ear? Sit the patient more upright to bring it down into view

Is it below the clavicle? Gently press in the RUQ (after asking about pain) for hepatojugular reflux

Remember the difference between the JVP and carotid pulsations

JVP	Carotid
More easily seen than felt	More easily felt than seen
Moves with posture/respiration	Static
Occluded with gentle pressure	Occluded only with firm pressure
Waveform: Vertical	Horizontal
Biphasic	Uniphasic

Features of an abnormal JVP

Giant systolic V waves	Tricuspid regurgitation (case 14)
Large diastolic A waves	Pulmonary hypertension
	Right-sided valvular stenosis
	AV dissociation (heart block/pacemaker malfunction)
Absence of A waves	Atrial fibrillation (case 7)
Non-pulsatile	
Rises with inspiration (Kussmaul's sign)	Restrictive cardiomyopathy/tamponade SVCO (case 28)

VIVA QUESTIONS

How would you monitor rheumatoid arthritis?

Rheumatoid arthritis is a systemic autoimmune disorder of unknown aetiology characterised by inflammatory, symmetrical small > large joint arthritis, pain, early morning stiffness, swelling and loss of function with destructive joint disease and ankylosis. Clinical monitoring is required with regard to symptoms/signs of active synovitis and functional impairment due to the destructive arthritis; this is supplemented by hand and foot radiographs to look for erosive disease evolution and serological markers of inflammation/rheumatoid factor titres.

Describe the rash that you may see in SLE

SLE is a chronic autoimmune disease affecting all races but with a predisposition for women and Black people. Impaired cellular immunity and exaggerated humoral immunity is seen, with production of autoantibodies to nuclear elements. The classic rash is a photosensitive erythematous rash in a butterfly distribution on the face.

What autoantibodies might you see in SLE?

Anti-nuclear antibodies are non-specific but present in 95%; anti-dsDNA antibodies are more specific. Anti-Smith, anti-phospholipid or other autoantibodies (eg Ro, La) may also be found.

What radiological changes do you see in multiple myeloma? What are the other cardinal features?

Myeloma is a plasma cell dyscrasia caused by a monoclonal expansion of plasma cells secreting monoclonal immunoglobulin. The characteristic radiological appearance of lytic lesions is rounded lucencies caused by osteoclast-activating factor produced by the infiltrating plasma cells. Radiodense expanded areas may occur due to collections of myeloma cells called plasmacytomas. Osteopenia/osteoporosis may also be present and predispose to fractures, especially vertebral.

The cardinal features are bone pain, vertebral fractures (loss of height/ spinal cord/root compression), symptomatic anaemia, immunoparesis with recurrent infections, renal failure and thrombocytopenia.

What are Osler's nodes and who was Osler?

Osler's nodes are the painful indurated areas on the pads of the fingers seen in bacterial endocarditis, resulting from immune complex deposition.

Sir William Osler was a Canadian-born physician who as a pathologist wrote the classic papers on hereditary haemorrhagic telangiectasia (Osler–Weber–Rendu syndrome), SLE and polycythaemia rubra vera. He was Physician-in-Chief at Johns Hopkins Hospital before becoming Regius Professor of Medicine at Oxford University.

What do you think of when you see a patient with clubbing?

Clubbing is increased curvature of the nails in all planes with obliteration of the nailfold angle and soft-tissue swelling. Mechanisms include the presence of vasodilators (eg right-to-left shunt preventing inactivation in the lung bed), activated platelets (eg chronic inflammation/infection – platelet-derived growth factor leads to increased vascular permeability, fibroblast proliferation and hyperplasia), increased growth hormone states and vagal mediation (eg clubbing in bronchial carcinoma may be reversed by vagotomy).

Causes can be grouped:

Chest	Chronic suppurative lung disease, fibrosis, carcinoma
Heart	Cyanotic heart disease, endocarditis
Gut	Cirrhosis, inflammatory bowel disease, coeliac disease
Endocrine	Acromegaly, thyroid acropachy

How would you treat acute gout?

Gout is a disorder of purine metabolism. The hyperuricaemia is due to over-production or under-secretion of uric acid (or both). This can be primary (eg enzyme abnormality, renal tubular defect) or secondary (eg increased production in lymphoproliferative disorders, reduced excretion due to thiazide diuretics). Uric acid is deposited in joints and other tissues. The acute arthritis usually affects the big toe.

Treatment is with NSAIDs for pain. Steroids may confer dramatic relief in refractory cases. Colchicine inhibits macrophage migration and phagocytosis of uric acid. Allopurinol may worsen acute gout – it confers prophylaxis by inhibiting xanthine oxidase, and hence urate production.

What are the radiological features of ankylosing spondylitis?

Ankylosing spondylitis is a chronic inflammatory disorder that predominantly affects the axial skeleton/sacroiliac joints and has a strong association with HLA-B27. The classic radiological finding is sacroiliitis as evidenced by erosions/sclerosis. Later, marginal syndesmophytes develop in the lumbosacral spine and 'squaring' of the vertebral body due to calcification of the interspinous ligaments gives the radiological 'bamboo spine'.

An asymmetrical large joint arthritis and enthesopathy (particuarly Achilles tendonitis/plantar fasciitis) can also occur.

Describe the typical symptoms of carpal tunnel syndrome

Compression of the median nerve at the wrist causes numbness, paraesthesia and pain in the median nerve distribution in the hand, although the patient often complains of whole hand numbness. Typically the symptoms are worse at night, waking the patient from sleep, and the patient vigorously shakes the hand to obtain relief. As progression occurs the patient begins to drop things and lose manual dexterity. The evolution of pain to sensory loss to wasting of the thenar eminence heralds end-stage nerve entrapment.

Tinel's test (tapping the median nerve over the carpal tunnel) reproduces/ worsens the symptoms.

SKIN

'Look at this patient's skin' or 'Examine this rash'

Skin diseases often cause confusion among students, mainly due to the extra terms that dermatologists use to describe lesions. To 'demystify' dermatology we think it is useful to describe a skin lesion as any surgical lump – this is something that should be second nature by the time of finals – and then use specific terms when needed.

The features of a lump that should be described are given below; some specific dermatological terms are also given. It is not necessary to use all these terms all the time but when used appropriately it shows a greater understanding on your part.

Colour	Erythema	Increased perfusion
Shape	Plaque	Flat-topped raised disc
	Macule	Flat area of discoloration
Size	Papule	<1 cm of elevated skin
	Nodule	>1 cm palpable mass
Surface	Vesicle	Blister <5 mm
	Bulla	Blister >5 mm
	Pustule	Blister containing pus
	Scale	Flaky keratin
	Crust	Dried exudate
Site	Exact position if localised	
	? Flexor/extensor surfaces if generalised	
	Unilateral/bilateral/symmetrical	

Edge

In the case of an ulcer you should describe the edge/base/depth/discharge/surrounding tissue.

There is no substitute for seeing lesions 'in the flesh', but also practise identifying and describing lesions with a colour atlas of dermatology, and go through how you would present the case if you saw it in the exam.

Systemic diseases that have cutaneous manifestations or dermatological conditions that have systemic complications are the commonest exam cases and you should be aware of these.

SKIN

Skin sign	Disease
Dermatitis herpetiformis	Coeliac disease (case 38)
Lupus pernio/nodules	Sarcoidosis (case 30)
Necrobiosis lipoidica (case 85)	Diabetes mellitus (case 53)
Pretibial myxoedema (case 84)	Graves' disease (case 55)
Erythema nodosum (case 82)	Many
Haemorrhagic telangiectasia (case 90)	GI bleeding (case 39)
Acanthosis nigricans	Neoplasia/diabetes/Cushing's disease
Vitiligo (case 88)	Many autoimmune diseases
Lupus rashes	SLE (case 64)/discoid lupus
Neurofibromatosis (case 80)	Systemic complications
Adenoma sebaceum	Tuberose sclerosis (epilepsy)
Port wine stain	Sturge–Weber syndrome (epilepsy – case 94)
Erythema multiforme (case 87)	Infections/drugs
Erythema ab igne (case 86)	Chronic pain – ? cause
Purpura/petechiae	Haematological disease / vasculitis/septicaemia
Xanthomas/xanthelasma	Hyperlipidaemia

Other common skin problems include:

Ulcers	Venous	
	Arterial	RA/sickle cell disease/PVD
	Neuropathic	Diabetes

Eczema/dermatitis (case 78)
Psoriasis (case 77)
Cellulitis (case 79)
Lichen planus   Itchy, thickened skin/Wickham's striae in mouth
Pityriasis rosea   Oval lesions on trunk/Herald patch
Pityriasis versicolor (case 89)
Rosacea   Facial papules/pustules/rhinophyma/telangiectasiae
    Eye blepharitis/conjunctivitis/uveitis
Shingles   Herpes zoster reactivation
Erythematous blistering rash in a dermatomal distribution/with pain

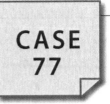

CASE 77 PSORIASIS

You may come across this when asked to examine either the rash or the hands. Invariably, one will lead to the other.

Introduce and expose

Observe   Generalised skin changes
              Scalp margins/'dandruff'

Hands   **Nails**   Pitting/ridging/onycholysis/hyperkeratosis/discoloration
           Skin   Plaques
                       Sausage-shaped fingers (dactylitis)

Joints   Five patterns: Rheumatoid-like (symmetrical small joint swelling)

                              Arthritis mutilans (highly destructive, telescoping of phalanges)

                              Ankylosing spondylitis like (sacroiliitis/spondyloarthropathy)

                              Mono-/oligoarthritis of large joints

                              DIP joint swelling/gross nail changes

Peripheries
           Elbow   Plaques
           Shin   Plaques
           Other sites Navel/natal cleft

The rash

Typical **salmon-pink** plaques with **silver-white** scale

Rarely

Flexural psoriasis in may be mistaken for eczema/intertrigo as scale may not be present

Guttate psoriasis typically follows a streptococcal upper respiratory tract infection, and presents as numerous small 'paint spot' lesions, usually on the trunk

Pustular psoriasis can affect the palms/soles of feet

Erythrodermic psoriasis affects almost the entire body, may be precipitated by abrupt treatment withdrawal, and is a dermatological emergency

COMMENT

Around 25% of patients with psoriasis will develop arthropathy, and most of these will have nail changes. Expect patients in examinations to have all three features (rash/nails/joints).

ECZEMA/ DERMATITIS

Atopy or contact allergies can cause a clinically indistinguishable picture.

Introduce and expose

Observe   Generalised skin changes
Well-demarcated, eg gloves, watch strap (allergy)

Hands   **Dry**/red/cracked skin, particularly between the fingers
Excoriations
Blistering/secondary infection (with crust)

Flexures   Anterior surface of wrist
Antecubital/popliteal fossae
Check behind the ears

Legs   'Venous eczema' (stasis dermatitis) over varicose veins

TREATMENT

Identify and avoid any precipitants
Moisturising creams – if it's dry, wet it
Steroid creams (weaker first)
Oral antihistamines for pruritus

If you are allowed to ask any questions, enquire about **asthma**/family history (atopic eczema) and any new detergent/hygiene products (contact dermatitis).

CELLULITIS

Differential diagnosis for a red, swollen leg should include cellulitis and DVT (case 5).

Introduce and expose

Wear gloves to examine wet rashes

Observe

Well/unwell

Rash

Hot/red/tender

Well demarcated/patchy

Swelling

Any site of injury (ulcer/trauma/Venflon site)

Any fluctuance/abscess/blistering

Crepitus/'bubble wrap' feel – necrotising fasciitis

Extras

Fever

COMMENT

Blood cultures/wound swabs are not always positive even with clinical cellulitis. Empirical treatment should cover common skin organisms (eg staphylococci/streptococci). Have a higher index of suspicion for MRSA with infected Venflon sites in inpatients.

Not systemically unwell	Consider oral flucloxacillin
Systemically unwell	Intravenous benzylpenicillin + flucloxacillin
Penicillin allergic	Erythromycin
MRSA suspected	Adjust to antibiotic sensitivities
Necrotising fasciitis	Clindamyin; early surgical input

NEURO-FIBROMATOSIS

Introduce and expose

Observe There may be very, very many skin lesions, and gross neurofibromatosis can be quite disfiguring

Skin lesions

Café-au-lait spots (more than five)

Axillary freckling

Neurofibromas (subcutaneous nodules/plexiform aggregation)

Mollusca fibrosa (pink cutaneous fibromas)

Skeletal

Kyphoscoliosis (50%)

Eyes Visual acuity may be decreased due to optic glioma

Lisch nodules ('freckling' of the iris due to hamartomas)

Fundoscopic changes

Hearing Decreased with acoustic neuroma

BP Increased if renal artery stenosis (intimal hyperplasia) or (more rarely) phaeochromocytoma

Neurological complications

Intracranial/intraspinal/peripheral nerve tumours

All types of tumour may occur (glioma/neuroma/meningioma/neurofibroma – 'a tumour soup')

The signs will depend on the location of the tumour

COMMENT

There are two types of neurofibromatosis, and both show autosomal dominant inheritance. This is complicated by a high spontaneous mutation rate (50% of cases are new mutations), and poor correlation between genotype and phenotype in neurofibromatosis 1 (NF1).

NF1   As described above

Also known as von Recklinghausen's disease

Chromosome 17

NF2   Bilateral acoustic neuromas

No skin/skeletal lesions

Other intracranial/intraspinal tumours common

Chromosome 22

DERMATOMYOSITIS/ POLYMYOSITIS

Introduce and expose

Usually female (twice as common as in men)

Observe Cachexia

Signs of other autoimmune connective tissue diseases

Hands **Nails** Rash around nail bed/nailfold infarcts

Skin Purple rash over knuckles (Gottron's papules)

Raynaud's phenomenon (case 68)

Face Heliotrope rash – purple/lilac rash of the eyelids (upper > lower) with swelling/puffiness

Other Purple rash over extensor surfaces (elbows/knees)

Proximal muscle weakness – ask the patient to stand from a low chair without using their arms

Muscle pain/tenderness

INVESTIGATIONS

ESR/CRP raised

Creatine kinase (CK) elevated

Autoantibodies if signs of mixed connective tissue disease

EMG (small, short motor unit potentials)

Muscle biopsy

TREATMENT

Oral steroids

Anti-rheumatics

COMMENT

Polymyositis is a related condition with muscle weakness and tenderness but without the skin changes.

Both conditions can overlap with other autoimmune connective tissue diseases, eg SLE, systemic sclerosis, Sjögren's syndrome, RA.

Both conditions are associated with malignancy (paraneoplastic syndromes), particularly upper GI/ovarian/breast/lung cancers. The overall incidence is 10–20%, but increases in older age.

ERYTHEMA NODOSUM

Site   Shins (occasionally thighs)

Description

Tender/red/smooth/shiny raised lesions

2–6 cm in diameter

Often follow a precipitating event by 2–6 weeks

Colour changes 'like a bruise' as the lesions resolve over 2–6 weeks

Causes   Sarcoidosis

Infection: classically streptococcal, TB, many others

Drugs: sulphonamides/penicillin/oral contraceptive

Inflammatory bowel disease

Pregnancy

Malignancy

Unknown/other

CASE 83

PYODERMA GANGRENOSUM

Site   Typically shins

Description

Ulcerating/necrotic/purulent spreading lesion

2–6 cm in diameter

Heals with scarring/poorly

Causes   Inflammatory bowel disease

Rheumatoid arthritis (including seronegative)

Haematological malignancies

Unknown

PRETIBIAL MYXOEDEMA

Site   Shins ± dorsum of feet

Description

Raised/waxy/purple–red lesions with 'orange-peel' appearance

Thickened skin with non-pitting, non-dependent oedema (severe cases)

Slow to resolve/may develop after treatment for underlying thyroid disease

Extras   Look for other signs of Graves' disease (exophthalmos)/goitre/thyroidectomy scar

Causes   Graves' disease (case 55)

Rarely, Hashimoto's thyroiditis (case 56)

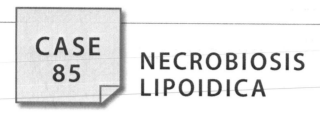

NECROBIOSIS LIPOIDICA

Site   Shins (occasionally arms), often bilateral

Description

Tender/raised/waxy/yellow plaque-like lesions with brown–red margins/nearby telangiectasia

Fragile, may ulcerate when injured

Can wax and wane

Heals poorly and with scarring

Extras   More common in women (with diabetes)

Look for other signs of diabetes:

Fingerprick BM testing scars/injection sites

Testing equipment/insulin by the bedside

Causes   Diabetes mellitus (case 53)

More common if microvascular complications, ie retinopathy/nephropathy

Rarely, rheumatoid arthritis (case 63)

COMMENT

Necrobiosis lipoidica diabeticorum can improve/resolve after transplantation, suggesting a possible immune cause.

ERYTHEMA AB IGNE

Site
Shins/lateral aspect of one leg (sat next to fire)
Low back/abdomen (hot water bottle)
Any site of chronic pain

Description
Pigmented/erythematous reticular discoloration
Can be blotchy/patchy
Skin may be atrophic/thin
Resolves well if identified early
Resolves poorly once pigmented (haemosiderin)

Causes
Chronic exposure to excessive heat:
Poor mobility (unable to move from fireside)
Poor thermoregulation (? hypothyroidism)
Application of heat packs/hot water bottles in chronic pain
(myeloma/osteoporosis)

ERYTHEMA MULTIFORME

Site   Extremities → trunk, usually symmetrical

Description

Multiple red papules/macules of various sizes, usually with pale centres ('target lesions')

Bullae can develop within lesions

Usually resolve over 7–10 days

Stevens–Johnson syndrome (erythema multiforme major) is a severe form:

   Widespread blistering/bullous rash

   Perioral predominance

   Orogenital ulceration

Causes   Often unknown (50%)

Herpes simplex infection

Mycoplasma pneumoniae

Drugs: most commonly sulphonamides/penicillin

Connective tissue diseases

Malignancy

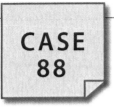

VITILIGO

Site   Anywhere, though commonly hands/face
            Usually symmetrical distribution

Description
            Patches of depigmentation with hyperpigmented border

Extras   Signs of other autoimmune diseases

Causes

Vitiligo is associated with many organ-specific autoimmune conditions, and more than one of the following may be present in the same individual. Ask for a family history of vitiligo/associated diseases.

            Alopecia areata/totalis
            Thyroid disease (hypo-/hyperthyroidism)
            Pernicious anaemia
            Addison's disease (case 58)
            Type 1 diabetes mellitus (case 53)
            Chronic active hepatitis
            Primary biliary cirrhosis

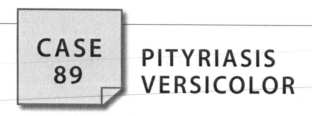

CASE 89

PITYRIASIS VERSICOLOR

Site   Anywhere, though commonly trunk/proximal limbs

Description

Patchy hypopigmentation (dark/sun-exposed skin)

Patchy hyperpigmentation (white/non-tanned skin)

Multiple small patches which can coalesce into large confluent regions

May be a fine scale

Reddens/darkens with heat/exercise

Causes   Pityrosporum yeast infection (*Malassezia* spp.)

This is usually a commensal on human skin and causes no problems in the vast majority of cases

Treatment

Selenium sulphide (anti-dandruff) shampoo

HEREDITARY HAEMORRHAGIC TELANGIECTASIA

Also known as Osler–Weber–Rendu syndrome. This case is often introduced to the candidate as the patient presented with anaemia (case 40) and/or a son/daughter/parent has the same problem (**autosomal dominant** inheritance)

Introduce and expose

Observe **Pallor** Blood loss (iron deficiency anaemia)

Lung – haemoptysis (bronchiectasis)

Gut – haematemesis/melaena

Nose – epistaxis

Telangiectasiae

Around the mouth/sun-exposed sites

Inside the mouth/on/under the tongue

Investigation for a source of GI blood loss may include upper/lower GI endoscopy and capsule endoscopy because anywhere in the tract may be affected

BULLOUS SKIN DISEASE

Pemphigoid and pemphigus present with large blisters (bullae).

Introduce and expose

Observe   More common with increasing age

Skin   Tense bullae, especially flexural surfaces (pemphigoid)
Flaccid bullae, which rupture easily and spread to adjacent skin with gentle pressure (pemphigus)
Painful oral mucosal lesions/ulcers (pemphigus)

In both cases, skin biopsy will confirm the diagnosis and treatment is with avoidance of infection and immunosuppression with steroids. Pemphigoid may require topical steroids only. Pemphigus is more severe and warrants systemic steroids ± other immunosuppressive agents.

VIVA QUESTIONS

What are the treatments for psoriasis?

Psoriasis is a chronic inflammatory skin disorder of unknown aetiology. Well-demarcated salmon-pink plaques with silvery scales are found on extensor areas, the scalp, navel and natal cleft. Symptomatic treatment is directed towards any pruritus and skin dryness (topical emollients), and reducing scale (keratolytics).

Topical treatment is with coal tar, steroids and calcipotriol (vitamin D_3 increases cell differentiation and reduces rash and scale). Systemic therapies include photochemotherapy with PUVA (psoralens and ultraviolet A), which is successful at clearing disease and delaying recurrence in chronic psoriasis.

Etretinate (vitamin A derived) and the folate antagonist methotrexate are used in severe disease unresponsive to other therapies. Steroids, hydroxycarbamide, colchicine and ciclosporin may also be helpful.

What is acanthosis nigricans, and when might you see it?

Acathosis nigricans is a dark (brown/black) diffuse 'velvety' pigmentation of the skin, classically in the axilla/skin folds. It may be congenital or associated with endocrine disorders (particularly thyroid disease, acromegaly, Cushing's disease and components of the metabolic syndrome, eg obesity, insulin resistance, polycystic ovarian syndrome) or malignancy (any, but particularly upper GI tumours).

What features of a pigmented skin lesion would make you suspicious of a malignant melanoma?

Any changes in a previously stable lesion would spark concern. Features that suggest higher risk include asymmetry, irregularity of border/surface/pigmentation, satellite areas of pigmentation, size (larger than the end of a pencil) and surface changes (itchiness/tenderness/bleeding/ulceration/erythema/scaling).

NERVOUS SYSTEM

Examination of the arm

You will seldom be asked to perform a full neurological examination due to time constraints.

Introduce and expose

Observe Wasting (especially small muscles of the hands)
Fasciculation (LMN lesions)

Arms outstretched

Pyramidal drift (UMN lesions)
Winging of the scapula (long thoracic nerve)

Tone Ask the patient to relax while you move his or her arms
Flexion/extension at the elbow – feel for 'clasp-knife'
Feel for supinator catch and cog-wheeling at the wrist

Power Test each in turn, always comparing the two sides

Movement	Root
Shoulder abduction	C5
Elbow flexion	C6
Elbow extension	C7
Wrist flexion	C7, C8
Wrist extension	C6, C7
Finger extension	C7
Finger spread	T1 (ulnar)
Thumb abduction	T1 (median)

Reflexes Demonstrate the biceps (C5), supinator (C6) and triceps (C7) jerks
Use reinforcement (jaw clench) before pronouncing a reflex absent
If reflexes brisk look for finger flexion jerks/ Hoffman's reflex (thumb flexion in response to tapping the distal third/fourth finger – UMN)

Sensation

>Light touch and pinprick (use a neuropin) – compare each dermatome C4–T2 on both sides
>
>Vibration at distal phalanx – if absent, move serially up until it is present (wrist/elbow/shoulder)

Coordination

>Finger–nose incoordination (hold your finger at arms' length) – no need to move your finger

Examination of the legs

Introduce and expose

Observe   Wasting/fasciculation

Pes cavus

Walking aids/splints/wheelchair

Tone   With the patient relaxed, gently roll the leg – the ankle should 'flop'

Flex the knee quickly – feel for a 'catch'

Check for ankle clonus by firmly dorsiflexing the foot and holding it up to feel the 'beats' of clonus against your hand: more than five beats is abnormal

Power   Test each in turn, always comparing the two sides

Movement	Root	Muscle
Hip flexion	L1, L2	Iliopsoas
Hip extension	S1	Glutei
Knee flexion	L5, S1	Hamstrings
Knee extension	L3, L4	Quadriceps
Ankle dorsiflexion	L4, L5	Tibialis anterior
Ankle plantarflexion	S1	Gastrocnemius

Reflexes   Demonstrate the knee (L3, L4) and ankle (S1) jerks

Use reinforcement (jaw clench/Jendrassik's manoeuvre) before pronouncing a reflex absent

Plantar responses (Babinski's sign) – use an orange stick

Sensation

Light touch (LT) and pinprick (PP – use a neuropin), compare each dermatome L2–S2 on both sides

LT alone is not always very helpful and sometimes confuses things; make sure that you know the main patterns of sensory loss (see below)

Vibration at distal phalanx – if absent, move serially up until it is present (medial malleolus/shin/knee/iliac crest/sternum)

Joint position sense (JPS) – use big toe on each side; if absent move up to larger joints (ankle/knee)

Temperature sensation is carried in the same tracts as PP, and can therefore be omitted

Coordination

Test for heel–shin ataxia

Tell the examiner 'At this stage I would usually go on to examine the back for scars, assess the gait and test for Romberg's sign'. Hopefully the examiner will stop you and ask you to present your findings.

Gait (case 106)

Ask the patient to walk a short way, turn around and walk back. Be sure to note:

Posture/arm swing/leg circumduction

Step size and equality

Foot drop

Ataxia

Romberg's sign

Ask the patient to stand with the feet together and eyes closed; stand nearby ready to prevent a fall

Positive if the patient sways/falls; this implies proprioceptive loss

Sensory patterns

Distal polyneuropathy ('stocking', PP > LT)

Dermatomal root lesions (PP ± LT)

Spinothalamic loss (PP but not JPS/vibration)

Dorsal column loss (JPS/vibration but not PP)

Examination of the cranial nerves

It is not usual to ask a candidate to examine all 12 cranial nerves and look at the fundi on one request. More commonly, you will be asked to look at the eyes (second, third, fourth and sixth nerves), examine the lower cranial nerves (fifth to twelfth but not sixth), or perform fundoscopy on a patient with dilated pupils (see case122). However, be prepared to start at the top and work down. It is important to look confident when testing the eyes and cranial nerves, so practise until you do.

I	Ask the patient 'Have you noticed any problems with your sense of taste or smell?' If the answer is yes, tell the examiner that you would usually go on to formally test these and see if the patient can breathe through each nostril

Eyes **Observe** Ptosis (case 118)
Nerve III/sympathetic/myasthenia
Squint (case 121)
Congenital/acquired
Exophthalmos (case 120)

II **Acuity**
Remember that visual acuity is the single most important aspect of vision
Ask 'Do you wear glasses/contact lenses?' – if yes, ask them to put them on
Tell the examiner 'I would like to test acuity formally with a Snellen chart at 6 m' – you may then be told the acuity; if not, test it with a full/pocket Snellen chart (if available – this looks more impressive than using your name badge)

Fields
Test against your own using a red neuropin. Do not forget to test for central scotoma

Pupils
Use a bright pen torch to test direct and consensual responses
Test accommodation by asking the patient to look at the far side of the room and then at your finger, held 10 cm from their nose. Make sure that you are able to see the pupillary response

Fundi

Usually a separate case, but state that you would like to examine the fundi after dilating the pupils. See case 122.

III, IV, VI Ask the patient to follow your pen torch with the eyes without moving the head, and to tell you if he or she sees double. Hold it vertically when testing horizontal movements and vice versa

Comment on which muscles are not working:

Lateral rectus (VI); superior oblique (IV)

Medial/superior/inferior rectus, inferior oblique (all III)

If it is not obvious when the patient complains of diplopia, cover one eye and ask which image disappears (the outermost image is from the affected eye, ie the one that has not moved)

If nystagmus is present describe which eye is affected the most and the direction of the fast phase (case 115)

Comment on internuclear ophthalmoplegia (116)

V **Motor**

Ask the patient to open the mouth (pterygoids) and then clench the teeth (masseter/temporalis)

Sensory

Check sensitivity to LT/PP over the three divisions (forehead/cheek/chin)

Tell the examiner 'I would like to test the corneal reflex' and if asked to do so use a wisp of sterile cotton wool. The afferent (sensory) limb is V^I, the efferent (motor) limb V^{II}

VII Assess the patient's facial movements by asking the patient to close the eyes tightly, raise the eyebrows, puff out the cheeks and show you the teeth

VIII	Ask the patient if they have any problems with hearing in either ear. A simple test is to rub the hair by the ear between your fingers, or whisper numbers

If a tuning fork examination is required, perform Weber's test (tuning fork on the vertex of the skull) and Rinne's test (tuning fork on the mastoid process)

Conductive: Weber's test lateralises to side of defect, and Rinne's test shows bone conduction to be better than air conduction – suggest that you would like to perform otoscopy

Sensorineural: Weber's test lateralises to the good side and Rinne's test is usually normal

It is important to test the hearing in any patient who has a nearby cranial nerve lesion (V/VII/IX/X) because a tumour compressing more than one nerve may be the underlying problem (case 130)

IX, X	Ask the patient to open the mouth and say 'Ah' Watch for palatal movement – the side that does not move is the abnormal one. Do not get into discussions about uvular movements; this only confuses the matter

Tell the examiner 'I would like to test the gag reflex in order to test sensation'. You won't usually be expected to do this, but you should know that the afferent (sensory) limb is IX and the efferent (motor) limb X

XII	Look at the tongue inside the mouth for wasting and fasciculation (LMN lesion), and then ask the patient to move it. A spastic tongue will not be wasted but will move slowly. Classically, the tongue will protrude to the side of weakness/paralysis

XI	Ask the patient to shrug the shoulders

Ask the patient to turn the head from one side to the other while you palpate the sternocleidomastoid muscles

CEREBROVASCULAR ACCIDENT

A cerebrovascular accident (CVA, or stroke) is defined as a sudden neurological deficit of vascular origin lasting longer than 24 hours. Resolution within 24 hours is a transient ischaemic attack (TIA).

PC   Asymmetrical weakness of a limb/limbs/face
Speech problems/sensory upset/visual disturbance
Collapse/headache but **not** blackout/syncope

HPC   **Onset sudden**
Course
          Static/Resolving/Progressing
History
          Previous TIAs/CVAs
          Amaurosis fugax
          Transient sensory/motor problems
Risk factors
          Smoking
          Hypertension
          Diabetes
          Hyperlipidaemia
Right or left handed?

PMH   Other vascular disease (IHD: angina; MI/PVD: claudication)
Atrial fibrillation (rheumatic heart/valve disease, MI)

FH   Increased vascular disease in family members

SH   Home House type/ground floor/stairs
                  Bathroom/bedroom upstairs/downstairs
                  Modifications (stairlift/commode/bath seat)
           Carers Relatives/friends/home help/dependants
           Allowances
           Mobility
                  Wheelchair/zimmer frame/sticks

DH   Antihypertensive medication
Aspirin/dipyridamole
Warfarin (may be the cause if haemorrhagic CVA)

ROS   Complications
Weight loss/swallowing difficulty
Constipation/bladder symptoms
Pneumonia (aspiration)/shoulder subluxation

EXAMINATION

General appearance
Plethoric/malar flush

CVS   BP/signs of hypertensive heart disease (pressure overload)
Atrial fibrillation (case 7)/heart murmurs
Carotid bruits

CNS   Dysphasia/dysarthria (case 134)
Apraxia
Sensory /visual inattention

Cranial nerves
Homonymous hemianopia (case 108)
UMN facial weakness (case 128)
Pseudobulbar palsy (case 133)

Peripheral nerves
Hemiparesis (spastic if old)
Unilateral UMN signs ± sensory loss
Increased tone/reflexes/clonus
Weakness without wasting
Decreased sensation/coordination
Upgoing plantars/positive Hoffman's sign

INVESTIGATIONS

BM   Exclude hypoglycaemia

ECG   Atrial fibrillation

CT of the brain

> Urgently if being considered for thrombolysis/
> depressed GCS (<13)/progressive symptoms/possible
> bleed (eg warfarin, neck stiffness/papilloedema/
> prominent headache)
>
> Otherwise within 24 h

TREATMENT

Acute CVA

Early diagnosis and imaging to confirm

Thrombolysis if:

> Haemorrhage excluded
>
> Within 3 hours of onset of symptoms
>
> Blood pressure less than 185/110 mmHg
>
> No contraindications (eg recent major bleed)

Aspirin 300 mg (unless contraindicated) for 2 weeks

Do not treat BP unless hypertensive emergency

Reverse anticoagulation if haemorrhagic CVA

Inpatient

Admit to a specialist acute stroke unit:

> Assess swallowing, nutrition
>
> Early mobilisation (sit up → sit out → get up → get out)

On discharge

Consider full anticoagulation after 2 weeks

Treat risk factors: antihypertensives, statins

TIA   Aspirin 300 mg ± dipyridamole

> Risk stratify to guide urgency of further investigations
>
> Carotid Doppler ultrasonography/ECG/echocardiography
>
> Consider early endarterectomy if >70% stenosis on side related
> to symptoms

COMMENT

Causes

Haemorrhagic	15%	Subarachnoid 5%/Intracerebral 10%
Ischaemic	85%	Thrombotic/embolic from the heart/carotids/ unknown 40%

Classification

Strokes may arise from the internal carotid (anterior) or vertebrobasilar (posterior) circulations. The Bamford classification is used to divide CVAs according to their territory, extent, and cause:

Total anterior circulation stoke (TACS) – all three of:

> Motor and sensory deficits in two-thirds of face/arm/leg
>
> Homonymous hemianopia
>
> Disturbance of higher function, eg dysphasia/neglect

Partial anterior circulation stroke (PACS)

> Any two of the above, or higher dysfunction alone, or more limited motor/sensory deficits

Lacunar stroke (LACS)

> Pure motor or pure sensory/ataxic hemiparesis

Posterior circulation stroke (POCS) – any of:

> Cranial nerve ± contralateral motor/sensory lesions
>
> Cerebellar signs/Brainstem signs
>
> Isolated homonymous hemianopia
>
> Bilateral sensory/motor deficit

The 'S' can be replaced with an 'I' for a confirmed infarct or 'H' for haemorrhage, eg a 'clinical' TACS becoming a CT-confirmed TACI.

CASE 93

MULTIPLE SCLEROSIS

The patient with MS is often young.

PC New/worsened neurological symptoms/weakness/disability (new diagnosis or relapse of known disease)
Problems due to established MS (urinary infection, respite)

HPC How and when did the patient first present?
Course of illness to date:
  If relapsing, number/frequency/nature of relapses
  If new diagnosis, any episodes before diagnosis of loss of vision in one eye (optic neuritis)/paraparesis with loss of continence (transverse myelitis)
Ascertain level of disability, if any, in the patient's 'steady state'
Enquire carefully about bladder symptoms:
  Urgency/urge incontinence/urinary infections
  Catheter/intermittent self-catheterisation/sheath
Infection/fever (may worsen disability/trigger relapse)
Fatigue is very common

PMH Obstetric history – relapses more common post partum

FH No clear inheritance, but about a ten times risk in first-degree relatives

SH This section of the history needs to be very thorough
Able to work/Invalidity benefit/Other allowances
Ambulant/wheelchair/able to transfer
Carers (family/social services)/district nurse/home help

DH Baclofen for spasticity/anticholinergics for incontinence
Intravenous steroids for recent relapse

EXAMINATION

MS, by its very nature, can produce a varied clinical picture. The following is an example.

General appearance is often normal

Depressed/anxious/euphoric

CNS Cerebellar dysfunction (staccato speech)

Cranial nerves

Optic atrophy (case 125) with relative afferent pupillary light:
Defect (Marcus–Gunn pupil)

Nystagmus (case 115)/internuclear ophthalmoplegia (case 116)
may be bilateral

Peripheral nerves

Spasticity legs > arms/clonus

Pyramidal weakness legs > arms

Brisk reflexes/finger flexion jerks/positive Hoffman's sign/
bilateral extensor plantars (easy to elicit)

Absent abdominal reflexes

Sensation affected in a patchy distribution/any modality

Finger–nose ataxia in arms

Gait – spastic and ataxic (case 106)

Urinalysis as urinary infection is common

INVESTIGATIONS

MRI of the brain   The best way to show white matter lesions

MRI of the spine   If presenting with cord symptoms

Visual evoked potentials Delayed (slow conduction in white
matter)

CSF   If diagnosis uncertain despite the above

90% will have oligoclonal bands

40% slight increase in protein concentration

30% slight increase in mononuclear cells

TREATMENT

Acute symptoms (new diagnosis/relapse)

High-dose corticosteroids for 3–5 days (speed recovery)

Specialist advice regarding other immunosuppressant therapies (eg azathioprine, intravenous immunoglobulin)

There is currently no treatment that has been conclusively shown to alter the course of the disease

Long-term treatment

Multidisciplinary team approach, especially physiotherapy and occupational therapy

Consider interferon-β for relapsing–remitting MS

Linoleic acid derivatives (eg sunflower oil)

Treatment for urinary frequency/incontinence

Prognosis

Favourable	Sensory symptoms/optic neuritis/young
Adverse	Progressive/incomplete recovery from initial attack
	Cerebellar ataxia/persistent weakness

COMMENT

MS affects the white matter of the CNS (brain/spinal cord) and not the peripheral nerves. By definition the patient must have at least two episodes (lesions) separated in both time and place (position within the CNS). MS can follow a number of different patterns:

> **Relapsing–remitting** is the case in 80% of new diagnoses. Periods of remission are interspersed with remissions

> **Secondary progressive** develops in 50% of patients with relapsing–remitting MS in the first 10 years. Relapses become more frequent, with incomplete remission and progression

> **Primary progressive** has gradual but continually worsening symptoms from the time of diagnosis (10–15% of patients)

Worsening of disability may be due to progression/relapse/intercurrent infection/unrelated disease.

Involvement of the optic nerve causes optic or retrobulbar neuritis. The characteristic clinical picture is of unilateral visual loss over hours to days associated with pain, especially on moving the eye. Colour vision is particularly affected. Recovery is the rule. In optic neuritis nerve head swelling is seen (papilloedema), whereas in retrobulbar neuritis nothing is seen (the patient sees nothing, the doctor sees nothing). Either can be followed by optic atrophy (case 125).

There are two unusual but very characteristic symptoms of MS:

1. **Uhthoff's phenomenon**: the effect of heat and exertion temporarily increases symptoms, most noticeably weakness of the legs/visual loss (inability to get out of a hot bath)

2. **Lhermitte's sign**: electric-shock- like sensations down the back and sometimes the thighs on bending the neck (can occur in other diseases involving the cervical spinal cord)

EPILEPSY

The key to diagnosing epilepsy is the history, both from the patient and where possible from a witness to the event.

PC   First fit/known epilepsy

HPC   Loss of consciousness (even if apparently awake)
            Loss of urinary continence
            Tongue biting
            Prodrome/onset/postictal confusion/drowsiness/paresis
            Precipitants – flashing lights, hyperventilation, sleep/lack of
            Partial seizures – psychic/cognitive phenomena/hallucinations
            in any sensory modality (olfactory, gustatory, auditory, visual,
            somatosensory)
            Limb jerking/rigidity – one area/spread/whole body
            Witness history, especially if fits/automatisms in sleep

PMH   Cerebrovascular disease/malignancy/brain injury

SH   Alcohol/drug use

DH   Antiepileptics – dose, regimen, compliance
            Any new drugs that may interfere with drug levels
            Drugs that lower seizure threshold (antibiotics, antipsychotics,
            aminophylline, many others)

EXAMINATION

General appearance is usually normal
            Port wine stain (Sturge–Weber syndrome)
            Tongue bite marks

CNS   May have postictal paresis (unilateral)

INVESTIGATIONS

Bloods including U&Es, calcium, glucose

Antiepileptic drug levels

ECG

CT	If suspicion of underlying cause of seizure
EEG	To support the diagnosis if epilepsy is suspected clinically – beware false-positives if history is poor Consider photic stimulation/hyperventilation/sleep
MRI	Especially if history/EEG suggests focal onset

TREATMENT

There is no need to start antiepileptic medication after a first fit as long as early referral to a specialist can be arranged. Most hospitals operate a 'first fit' clinic with investigations and first consultation with a specialist within 2 weeks.

Education for the patient and carers

Contact with a specialist epilepsy service (specialist nurse)

Antiepileptics guided by type of seizure:

Sodium valproate may be used for all patterns

Carbamazepine for partial/tonic–clonic seizures

Newer agents, eg lamotrigine, if not tolerated

Levetiracetam/clobazam as second-line/adjuncts

Women of childbearing age – advice on contraception and antiepileptic drugs in pregnancy and breastfeeding

Surgery may be considered for focal seizures

Vagus nerve stimulation (refractory cases)

Stop driving for 6 months after a first fit (5 years for LGVs/PCVs)

Epileptic emergencies

Prolonged seizures (>5 min) or recurrent (more than three in an hour)

Rectal diazepam (10–20 mg; may be repeated once)

Referral to hospital

Status epilepticus (seizure >30 min or <30 min between seizures)
    ABCDE approach (see case 144)
    Intravenous lorazepam (4 mg; may be repeated once)
    Intravenous phenytoin infusion
    Propofol/thiopental if refractory – call an anaesthetist

COMMENT

In **simple partial** seizures consciousness is unaffected and positive sensory/neuropsychiatric phenomena are usually predominant.

Complex partial seizures have impairment of consciousness, and often automatisms such as lip-smacking or purposeless walking.

Either can go on to become a **secondary generalised** seizure.

Primary generalised seizures may be absences (petit mal), myoclonic, clonic, tonic, **tonic–clonic** (grand mal) or atonic.

CASE 95   HEADACHE

There are often few physical findings on examination. Therefore a thorough history is essential to reach an accurate diagnosis.

PC	Pain	In the morning/when bending/straining (raised ICP)
		Bilateral, band-like (tension)/unilateral (most others)
		Scalp tenderness/jaw claudication (GCA)
		Facial pain (trigeminal neuralgia)
		Timing: sudden, severe (SAH)/cluster headache/after fall/trauma (subdural)
	Aura/visual disturbance (migraine)	
	Photophobia/vomiting (meningitis/migraine/SAH)	
	Odd behaviour (encephalitis)	
HPC	Exposure to: carbon monoxide, nitrates, calcium-channel blockers	
	Withdrawal from: alcohol, opioids, oestrogens, corticosteroids, TCAs, SSRIs, NSAIDs	
	Constitutional symptoms (brain primary/secondary cancer)	
	Exertional onset (SAH)/during coitus (coital cephalgia)	
PMH	Cancer (metastatic brain cancer)	
	Polymyalgia rheumatica (GCA)	
	Angina (exposure to nitrates may produce headache)	
	Depression, insomnia, anxiety (tension)	
FH	Close contact has become unwell (meningitis)	
	Familial tendency (migraines/SAH with polycystic kidneys)	
DH	Anticoagulants/alcoholism (subdural haematoma)	
	Chronic analgesics: codeine, paracetamol, NSAIDs, triptans	
ROS	GI upset/teichopsia/fortification spectra (migraine)	
	Limb–girdle pain/weakness (GCA)	
	Blurred/altered vision (raised ICP)/amaurosis fugax (GCA)	
	Transient visual loss (IIH)	

SH Caffeine/alcohol/dietary precipitants (chocolate, cheese)
Smoking (migraine, metastatic cancer, SAH)

EXAMINATION

General appearance

Overweight (IIH)/cachexia (malignancy)
Photophobia (meningitis/SAH)
Hypertension/fever/signs of sepsis/drowsiness
Painful scalp on palpation (GCA, trigeminal neuralgia)
Lacrimating red eye (cluster)
Kernig's sign/pain on straight-leg raise; non-blanching rash/
cool peripheries; painful legs (meningitis)

Fundoscopy and visual field examination

INVESTIGATIONS

FBC Polycythaemia (cause)/anaemia (eg malignancy)
U&Es/calcium (dehydration)/blood sugar/TFTs
CRP/ESR raised in infection/GCA (temporal artery biopsy)
ECG can have acute changes in intracranial bleed
CT of the head/lumbar puncture, eg for meningitis/SAH/IIH

TREATMENT

If meningitis is suspected, give intravenous benzylpenicillin before urgent transfer to hospital. Third-generation cephalosporins are the empirical treatment before causative organisms are identified.

Lifestyle changes, trigger avoidance:

GCA	Prednisolone 40 mg a day until symptoms resolve then gradual reduction/if visual symptoms, 60 mg and urgent referral to ophthalmology
Migraine	Simple analgesia (NSAIDs) ± antiemetic If no relief then triptans or ergotamine
Cluster	Treat cluster with high-flow O_2, sumatriptan Prophylaxis with prednisolone, verapamil
Tension	Simple analgesia – avoid chronic use
Neuralgia	Neuropathic painkillers – antiepileptics/TCAs
SAH	Nimodipine 60 mg 4-hourly; urgent referral
Raised ICP	Treat cause, eg radiotherapy; therapeutic lumbar puncture/shunt (IIH); rarely craniotomy

COMMENT

Tension headache is the most common. Pain is typically in a band-like distribution around the head, has a gradual onset, is less severe than migraine with no associated symptoms, and generally responds to analgesics.

Typical symptoms of raised ICP include pain, vomiting and visual blurring. On fundoscopy the optic disc may be blurred. Causes include intracranial masses, bleeding or idiopathic ('benign') intracranial hypertension (IIH). CT before lumbar puncture is mandatory.

Migraine may or may not be preceded by an aura, which is commonly visual, in the form of either flashing lights or fortification spectra. Headache, nausea and vomiting may follow. Headaches are commonly unilateral and severe, often with photophobia.

Temporal arteritis (GCA) typically affects people over the age of 50, with women affected two to three times more commonly than men; 50% of patients will also have polymyalgia rheumatica. The disease must be treated aggressively because of the risk of permanent visual loss.

Trigeminal neuralgia can affect any of the divisions of the trigeminal nerve, although most commonly the maxillary or mandibular branches. Pain is usually a brief, sharp, stabbing, shock-like pain that can be brought on by touch, eg combing the hair.

Cluster headaches are unilateral and are localised around or behind the eye. The sharp, excruciating pain comes on rapidly, without aura, and lasts from 45 min to 90 min. The headaches commonly occur within 2 h of falling asleep, with periods of remission between clusters of attacks. Ipsilateral lacrimation or nasal discharge is often present.

Analgesia-associated headache is present for 15 or more days a month and develops or worsens while taking regular painkillers. Any simple analgesia may be the cause, but compound medications are more likely to cause symptoms. Withdrawal of analgesics is the treatment.

SAH is associated with a thunderclap headache (sudden onset, worst pain ever), often in the occipital area.

CO poisoning may present as a headache with irritability, nausea, weakness, tachycardia and tachypnoea. The classic rosy-pink appearance associated with carboxyhaemoglobin is rarely seen before death. Remove the patient from the source of CO and give high-flow O_2.

PARKINSON'S DISEASE

You should be happy to have a case of Parkinson's disease (PD) in the exam because the signs are easy to elicit and should be familiar. You may be asked to approach the patient in several ways: examine the gait (case 106)/upper limbs/speech/lower cranial nerves (facial expression).

Introduce and expose

Observe	Poor posture (stooping/slumped in chair)
	Slow shuffling gait/reduced arm swing/poor balance
	Quiet monotonous speech/pauses
Face	Lack of facial expression/drooling of saliva
	Glabellar tap does not habituate as in normal

Arms	**Bradykinesia (slow)**	Moving thumb to other fingers
	Rigidity (stiff)	Best demonstrated in the wrist
	Tremor (shaky)	'Pill rolling'
		At rest/often asymmetrical
		Reduced on movement
		Brought out by motor distraction – ask the patient to raise and lower one arm while you watch the other for increased tremor

COMMENT

L-Dopa treatment may lead to chorea/dystonic movements, especially of the hands and feet. In contrast with tremor these movements increase during action.

You should be aware of the Parkinson's plus syndromes:

Multisystem atrophy (MSA/Shy–Drager syndrome) is Parkinson's disease with cerebellar ataxia and autonomic neuropathy

Progressive supranuclear palsy (PSP/Steele–Richardson–Olszewski syndrome) is Parkinson's disease with ophthalmoplegia, and at later stages pseudobulbar palsy and dementia

Dementia with Lewy bodies is a clinical overlap between Parkinson's and Alzheimer's diseases

MOTOR NEURONE DISEASE

Motor neurone disease (MND) is notable in exams for the mixture of upper and lower motor neurone signs, and the absence of sensory signs and bladder symptoms.

Introduce and expose

Observe

Wasting, especially of the small muscles of the hand/foot

Fasciculation (tongue and/or limbs)

Tone   Normal or increased (spastic)

Power   Either segmental (LMN) or pyramidal (UMN) weakness

Reflexes

Exaggerated (usually)/diminished/absent

Sensation

Normal

Coordination

Normal

Extras   Bulbar (case 132)/pseudobulbar (case 133) palsies

COMMENT

Cause	Unknown (90%)/familial (10%)
Pathology	Degeneration of:
	Anterior horn cells/corticospinal tract
	Motor cortex/cranial nerve nuclei/corticobulbar tract
Typically	Age 45–65/males > females/median survival 3 years

Classification

Various names are given to various clinical presentations of MND:

Progressive muscular atrophy with isolated LMN signs

Progressive lateral sclerosis with isolated UMN signs

Amyotrophic lateral sclerosis with mixed signs, also known as Lou Gherig's disease after a famous US baseball player who had the disease

Bulbar or **pseudobulbar palsy** in isolation may be caused by MND

MYOTONIC DYSTROPHY

You should be able to recognise the characteristic facial appearance.

Introduce and expose

The patient may find it hard to release the handshake

Observe **Myopathic facies**

Snarl/poor smile/looks sad

Drooping mouth/probably unable to whistle

Frontal balding

Temporal wasting

Ptosis (case 118) Unilateral/bilateral

Cataracts

Thick 'coke bottle' glasses

Other features

Myotonia	Slow relaxation of muscles
	Difficulty releasing grip (worse in cold conditions)
Weakness	Especially forearms
Reflexes	Decreased
Low IQ	
Endocrine	Insulin resistance (type 2 diabetes mellitus)
	Small testes
	Goitre (case 74)
Cardiac	Conduction defects

Inheritance

Autosomal dominant/more often identified in men

Triplet repeat – shows anticipation (increased severity with each generation)

COMMENT

It is important that anaesthetists are aware of this condition preoperatively.

MYASTHENIA GRAVIS

Introduce and expose

Observe **Myopathic facies**
Snarl/poor smile/looks sad
Drooping mouth/probably unable to whistle
Ptosis (case 118) Bilateral/asymmetrical/fatigable
May have compensatory 'lid retraction' due to frontalis activity on the stronger side
Eye movements
Variable strabismus (case 121) (diplopia does not fit a single nerve lesion)

	Fatigable
Voice	Weak
Airway	Poor swallow
Breathless if very severe (unlikely in an exam)	
Muscle weakness	Proximal > distal
Reflexes	Normal

No sensory signs

Extras Associated with other autoimmune diseases
Thymoma/thymic hyperplasia

This is an autoimmune disease of the neuromuscular junction and may present in the exam for several reasons.

Myasthenia may be confined to the eyes with a combination of ptosis, ophthalmoplegia and diplopia (similar to thyroid eye disease but with ptosis and no exophthalmos). In addition, myasthenia shows fatigability. If you ask the patient to keep looking up the ptosis will worsen. Generalised myasthenia is not common but again fatigability is the hallmark.

Do not confuse myasthenia gravis and the Lambert–Eaton myasthenic syndrome. The latter is usually associated with small-cell lung cancer, more prominently affects the proximal muscles, reflexes are reduced/absent and contraction strength increases with repeated stimuli.

CASE 100 SYRINGOMYELIA

Rare in real life – disproportionately common in exams!

Introduce and expose

Observe Puffy cyanosed hands
Wasting, especially small muscles of the hand
Scars (from painless burns/injuries)
Charcot's joints   Elbow/shoulder

Tone

Power Segmental (LMN) weakness – most marked distally
Pyramidal (UMN) weakness below syrinx (legs)

Reflexes Absent in upper limbs (LMN)
Brisk in lower limbs (UMN – pyramidal tract damage)

Sensation
Dissociated/suspended (normal above and below):
Loss of pain and temperature sensation (crossing spinothalamic fibres)
Preserved light touch/joint position sense/vibration (uncrossed dorsal column fibres)
Impaired pain/temperature sensation in hands/arms/'shawl' distribution over shoulders/upper back

Coordination
Normal

Extras Pain   Neck/shoulders/radicular down arms

COMMENT

Differential

> Syrinx (a fluid-filled cavity within the spinal cord)
>
> Central cord tumour

Associations

> Arnold-Chiari malformation (?downbeat nystagmus)
>
> Hydrocephalus
>
> Horner's syndrome (case 112)
>
> Kyphoscoliosis
>
> Spastic paraparesis (case 101)

Syringobulbia refers to syrinx formation in the brainstem giving rise to cranial nerve lesions.

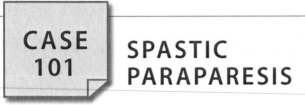

CASE 101

SPASTIC PARAPARESIS

Introduce and expose

Observe Disuse atrophy/contractures – implies long standing
Fasciculation (MND – case 97)

Tone Increased in legs (**spasticity**)
Ankle and patellar clonus

Power Leg weakness Flexors > extensors
The weakest movements are hip flexion,
knee flexion and ankle dorsiflexion

Reflexes Brisk knee and ankle jerks
Extensor plantars

The examiner may stop you here – otherwise:

Sensation
Look for a **sensory level** on the trunk (pinprick)

Coordination
Difficult to assess in presence of spasticity/weakness

Gait Stiff awkward, 'scissors' gait

Extras Urinary/faecal incontinence

COMMENT

Causes

1. Spinal cord compression: the most important to exclude – check for a sensory level. Consider cervical spondylosis in elderly patients/collar

2. **Multiple sclerosis** (case 93): especially younger patients

3. **Motor neurone disease** (case 97)

4. Syringomyelia (case 100)

5. Syphilis (case 114)

6. Subacute combined degeneration of the cord (vitamin B_{12})

7. Spinal cord infarction

8. Familial spastic paraparesis

9. Parasagittal lesions

10. Bilateral cerebrovascular disease

There are many other rarer causes.

Remember that paraparesis is a weakness of both lower limbs. If the arms are involved as well, the correct term is 'quadriparesis', which implies a higher (cervical) lesion.

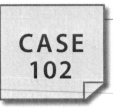

CASE 102   MYOPATHY

Introduce and expose

Observe   Wasting **proximal** > distal

Tone   Normal

Power   Weakness **proximally**
> Hip flexion/extension weak
> Ankle dorsiflexion/plantarflexion normal
> Difficulty getting out of a low chair without using hands/armrests

Reflexes   **Usually normal** (may be depressed)
> Flexor plantars

Sensation
> **Normal**

Coordination
> Normal – within the limits of the weakness

Gait   **'Waddling'**
> Unable to rise from crouching position

COMMENT

Causes Inflammatory myopathies

Polymyositis/dermatomyositis (case 81)

Inclusion body myositis

Metabolic/endocrine myopathies

Cushing's syndrome (case 57)

Hyper-/hypothyroidism (cases 55 and 56)

Muscular dystrophies (= genetic myopathies)

Duchenne's/Becker's dystrophy

Myotonic dystrophy (case 98)

Polymyalgia rheumatica (GCA)

Paraneoplastic

Lambert–Eaton myasthenic syndrome (see case 99)

Remember, myopathies are **proximal** (except myotonic dystrophy), and peripheral neuropathies are **distal** (except Guillain–Barré syndrome).

Other causes of hip flexor weakness may be misdiagnosed if care is not taken. Be sure that the weakness is not the result of pyramidal disease (case 92) or diabetic femoral amyotrophy (case 53).

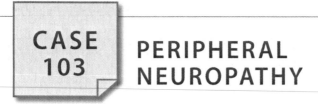

CASE 103

PERIPHERAL NEUROPATHY

Introduce and expose

Observe   Distal muscle wasting (especially peroneal)/foot drop
Pes cavus/claw toes
Charcot's joints
Callus formation/skin ulceration (especially under metatarsal heads)
Foot drop splint at side of bed

Tone   May be flaccid if severe weakness

Power   Distal weakness (ankle dorsiflexion/plantarflexion/inversion/eversion)
Eventually also weakness in hands

Reflexes   **Absent ankle jerks** (remember reinforcement)
Knee jerks absent/depressed

Sensation
Loss of pinprick and light touch in a (glove) and 'stocking' distribution (feet earlier than hands):
'Patchy loss to pinprick more marked distally consistent with a peripheral neuropathy'
Loss of **vibration** sense to ankles/knees/iliac crests/sternum
Loss of JPS at toes

Coordination

Gait   If foot drop is prominent patient may be seen to lift feet up high before they return them to the ground with a 'slap' (case 106)

Romberg's
Should be positive if you found JPS impaired

Extras   Suggest examining the upper limbs for similar signs and ask to examine the urine (diabetes)
Thickened nerves (rare)

COMMENT

When testing sensation, first test pinprick on the thigh, where it will be sharp, then move to the foot. Ask the patient (with their eyes shut) to report when the sensation changes as you move up the leg. Repeat on the medial and lateral aspects of the leg. Repeat on the other leg.

Causes

There are many causes, the most common being:

MADD – **m**alignancy/**a**lcohol/**d**iabetes/**d**rugs

A useful summary is ABCDEFGH:

> **A**lcohol/amyloid
>
> **B** vitamin deficiencies
>
> **C**onnective tissue diseases/cancer (but say neoplasia!)
>
> **D**iabetes/drugs
>
> **E**verything else!
>
> **F**riedreich's ataxia
>
> **G**uillain–Barré syndrome
>
> **H**ereditary motor sensory neuropathy
> (HMSN = Charcot–Marie–Tooth disease)

In 40% no cause is identified, despite full investigation.

PES CAVUS

Introduce and expose

Observe   High-arched feet
Clawing of the toes
Associated distal muscular atrophy

Causes   Idiopathic
Familial
Long-standing neuropathies (case 103)
HMSN (Charcot–Marie–Tooth disease)
Friedreich's ataxia
Syringomyelia
Spina bifida
Old polio (more likely if pes cavus is unilateral)

ABSENT ANKLE JERKS, EXTENSOR PLANTARS

This one is an 'old chestnut' brought out for exams.

If you find absent ankle (and possibly knee) jerks you will almost certainly be asked for possible causes. The pathophysiology is:

A **Damage to the monosynaptic reflex arc** and therefore reflex loss (peripheral nerve/dorsal root ganglion/α-motor neurone)

B **Damage to the corticospinal tract** leading to an extensor plantar

Causes

1. Subacute combined degeneration of the cord

Cause	Vitamin B$_{12}$ deficiency (pernicious anaemia)
Pathology	Demyelination of white matter in cord and peripheral nerve
Typically	Patient in 60s/fair hair/blue eyes/pallor (macrocytic anaemia)

2. Friedreich's ataxia

Cause	Autosomal recessive (onset <20 years)
	Autosomal dominant (onset >20 years)
Pathology	Degeneration of dorsal columns/corticospinal tracts/cerebellum (case 107)/spinocerebellar tracts/dorsal root ganglia/peripheral nerves

3. Motor neurone disease

4. Syphilitic taboparesis

5. Combination of two common conditions: probably the common scenario, eg elderly patient with cervical spondylosis (extensor plantars) and diabetic neuropathy (absent ankle jerks)

6. Structural lesion at the conus: the conus is the terminal part of the spinal cord (at the level of the T12–L1 vertebral bodies). Within the spinal canal at this point there are many nerves passing downwards before leaving through their appropriate foramina. A lesion within the canal at this level will therefore damage both upper and lower motor neurones.

GAIT ABNORMALITIES

If you are asked to examine the gait there are only a few possibilities. Once you have recognised the pattern, ask to elicit other signs to confirm your diagnosis.

Spastic   The patient walks with hyperextended lower limbs using a scissor-like action/'walking through treacle'. Due to UMN lesions affecting both legs (case 101)

Hemiparesis

One leg is held extended, often with foot drop. The leg is swung out (circumducted) to avoid tripping. Due to UMN lesion of one side.

Isolated foot drop

Common peroneal nerve palsy

Cerebellar

Broad-based gait often falling to one side (case 107)

Sensory ataxic

'Foot slapping' gait due to loss of proprioception, usually from neuropathy (case 103)/dorsal column loss (vitamin B_{12} deficiency/syphilis). The patient will have to look at the ground to compensate for proprioceptive loss

Parkinsonian

Unsteady/small steps/shuffling

Difficult to start/festinant (accelerating)/difficult to stop/difficult to turn (unsteady)

No arm swing (case 96)

Waddling

Seen with myopathies (muscular dystrophy, proximal muscle weakness) due to the loss of control of the pelvis while one leg is off the floor (case 102)

CEREBELLAR SYNDROME

You may be asked to examine for cerebellar signs, or on finding one be asked to go on and look for more.

There are groups of signs to look for. From the top down:

Nystagmus (case 115)
>   Lesion is ipsilateral to the fast phase

Dysarthria
>   **Ataxic** 'staccato' speech – ask the patient to say 'British constitution'

Ataxia (finger–nose)
>   Ipsilateral to lesion
>   Past-pointing (dysmetria)

Dysdiadochokinesis
>   Poor rapid alternating movements

Ataxia (heel–shin)

Gait   Broad based, falls to the side of lesion

A useful acronym is **DANISH** (**d**ysdiadochokinesis, **a**taxic gait, **n**ystagmus, **i**ntention tremor, **s**taccato speech, **h**ypotonia).

Causes	Demyelination	MS (case 93)
	Vascular	Posterior circulation stroke (case 92)
	Tumour	In posterior fossa (primary/secondary)
	Degenerative	Paraneoplastic (eg case 25)
		Alcohol excess (case 139)
		Hypothyroidism (case 56)
		Friedreich's ataxia (case 103)
	Drug toxicity	Phenytoin/carbamazepine
		Idiopathic/primary

HOMONYMOUS HEMIANOPIA

Introduce and expose

Observe Look for signs of ipsilateral hemiparesis, eg right homonymous hemianopia (HH)/right-sided UMN facial palsy/right-sided weakness (unable to shake hands, etc)

Acuity Normal

Fields Lesion **posterior to the optic chiasm** (see p. 181)

Optic tract	May be asymmetrical	
Optic radiation	Upper quadrants	Temporal
	Lower quadrants	Parietal
Occipital cortex	? Macular sparing	

Pupils Normal

Movements
Normal

Fundi Normal/papilloedema if space-occupying lesion

Extras Tell the examiner you would like to go on to look for other focal neurological signs, especially those commonly found in CVAs (ipsilateral hemiparesis)/neglect with left HH/dysphasia with right HH

INVESTIGATIONS

Formal perimetry

CT of the brain

Risk factors for CVA:

BP (hypertension)

BM stix (diabetes)

ECG (atrial fibrillation)

Carotid Doppler ultrasonography (TIAs)

Causes

Most cases are the result of cerebrovascular disease. Tumours and other space-occupying lesions are less common.

BITEMPORAL HEMIANOPIA

Introduce and expose

Observe May be signs of pituitary disease (cases 59 and 60)

Acuity Normal unless coexisting pressure on optic nerves

Fields Lesion **at the optic chiasma** (see p. 181) causing damage to crossing nasal retinal fibres (temporal fields)
Upper quadrant = inferior fibres = ? pituitary
Lower quadrant = superior fibres = ? craniopharyngioma

Pupils Normal

Movements
Normal

Fundi Optic atrophy if coexisting pressure on optic nerves

Causes Pituitary tumour   Look for abnormal pituitary function
– although many macroadenomas are non-secretory/ asymptomatic
Craniopharyngioma/meningioma/aneurysm

CENTRAL SCOTOMA

There is a large overlap between this and optic atrophy (case 125).

Introduce and expose

Observe

Acuity   Decreased

Fields   Loss of **centre of visual field** with preservation of peripheral field

Pupils   Normal/may have relative afferent pupillary defect (Marcus–Gunn pupil, more constriction to consensual than direct light reflex)

Movements   Normal

Fundi   Depends on cause: Optic atrophy (case 125)
                                       Macular disease

Causes

Primary   Damage to nerve
                Demyelination (case 93)
                Compression (glaucoma/tumour/Paget's disease (case 70)/thyroid eye disease (case 120))
                Ischaemic
                Toxic (methanol/lead/quinine)
                Infective (syphilis)
                Nutritional (vitamin B_{12} deficiency)
                Hereditary (Friedreich's ataxia (case 103)/Leber's optic atrophy)

Secondary   To chronic papilloedema (case 126)

Consecutive To retinal disease
                Retinitis pigmentosa (case 127)
                Choroiditis

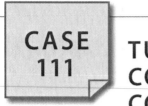

CASE 111

TUNNEL VISION/ CONCENTRIC CONSTRICTION

Introduce and expose

Observe ? Syndromic appearance (retinitis pigmentosa)
Hearing aid (Usher's syndrome)

Acuity Normal
May have night blindness (loss of rods)
Decreased if advanced disease

Fields Loss of **peripheral fields** with normal central field

Pupils Normal

Movements
Normal

Fundi Retinitis pigmentosa (case 127)
Cupping of optic disc in glaucoma (? optic atrophy)
Choroidoretinitis
Papilloedema (case 126) – also increased size of blind spot

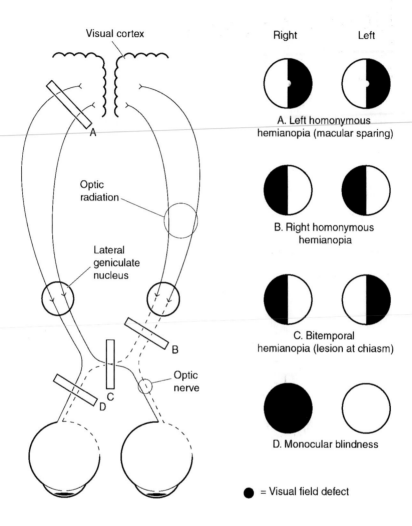

Visual cortex

Optic
radiation

Lateral
geniculate
nucleus

Optic
nerve

A

B

C
D

Right   Left

A. Left homonymous
hemianopia (macular sparing)

B. Right homonymous
hemianopia

C. Bitemporal
hemianopia (lesion at chiasm)

D. Monocular blindness

● = Visual field defect

Figure 1

HORNER'S SYNDROME

Caused by damage to the sympathetic nervous system (oculosympathetic palsy).

Introduce and expose

Observe   Ptosis (case 118)/enophthalmos/hypohidrosis

Acuity   Normal

Fields   Normal

Pupils   Small (**miosis**)
Reacts to light and accommodation

Movements
Nystagmus (case 115) if brainstem disease

Fundi   Normal

Extras   Eyes
Heterochromia of iris (less pigment in affected eye)
Neck
Lymphadenopathy/scars/carotid aneurysm/ipsilateral carotid bruit (dissection of artery)
Lung
Apical 'Pancoast's' tumour (T1 muscle wasting and sensory loss – case 73)
Brainstem
CVA (case 92)/MS (case 93) /
Syringomyelia (case 100)
Look for nystagmus (case 115)/bulbar palsy (case 132)/ sensory loss
Idiopathic in young women

COMMENT

This is an examiners' favourite and you should be aware of the anatomical course of the sympathetic supply of the pupil:

Midbrain → medulla → T1 cord → T1 root → thoracic ganglion → ascending preganglionic fibres → carotid plexus → long ciliary nerve → short ciliary nerve → radial pupillodilator muscle/muscle of Müller.

The classic clinical triad is **ptosis, miosis, anhidrosis.**

Think 'Little Jack Horner' for a small pupil with a sunken eye.

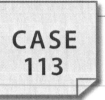

CASE 113

HOLMES–ADIE PUPIL

Caused by damage to the parasympathetic nervous system.

Introduce and expose

Observe   Young female

Acuity   Normal

Fields   Normal

Pupils   Unilaterally **dilated** (regular)
Very **slow reaction** to light and slow returning to normal
Slow reaction to accommodation

Movements
Normal (compare nerve III lesion – the major differential)

Fundi   Normal

Extras   Decreased/absent ankle jerks
Constricts with dilute methacholine (normal pupils do not) –
implies denervation hypersensitivity

COMMENT

This is a benign condition.

Other causes of a dilated pupil:

> Nerve III palsy (ptosis/eye looks 'down and out')
>
> Eyedrops (tropicamide/atropine)
>
> Drugs – cocaine, opiate withdrawal

Causes of a small pupil:

> Old age
>
> Horner's syndrome (case 112)
>
> Argyll Robertson pupil (case 114)
>
> Disease in the pons (CVA, etc)
>
> Eyedrops (pilocarpine)
>
> Drugs – opiates (especially toxicity)

ARGYLL ROBERTSON PUPIL

Traditionally caused by syphilis, although the mechanism is unclear. When suggesting this as a differential diagnosis in front of a patient, call it *Treponema pallidum*.

Introduce and expose

Observe   Bilateral ptosis (frontalis overactivity may overcome this)

Acuity   May be decreased if diabetes is the cause

Fields   Normal

Pupils   **Small, irregular**
No response to light/normal accommodation
'Accommodates but doesn't react' – the prostitute's pupil

Movements
Normal

Fundi   Optic atrophy (syphilis)/diabetic fundus (diabetes)

COMMENT

Causes   Neurosyphilis/diabetes/pinealomas
Ask to check treponema serology and urine glucose

Argyll Robertson pupil = accommodation reflex preserved

Neurosyphilis may occur in several different patterns

Meningovascular
A vasculitis that may affect any part of the CNS

Tabes dorsalis   Dorsal column loss:
Loss of joint position sense
Loss of vibration sense
Loss of deep pain sensation
Broad-based gait/high stepping
Charcot joints
Bladder insensitivity
Lightning pains/hypotonia

General paresis of the insane (GPI)
Dementia/fits/tremor (lips/tongue)

Taboparesis
Tabes dorsalis and GPI with additional UMN signs (pyramidal weakness/extensor plantars)

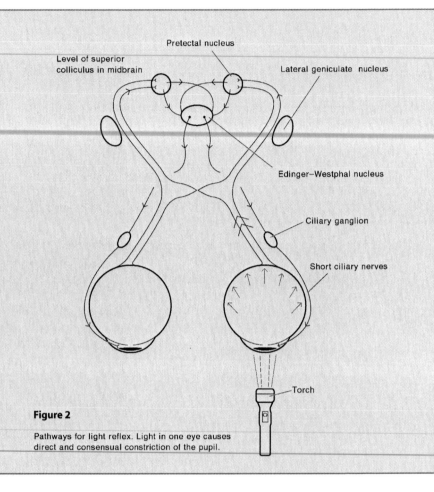

Pretectal nucleus

Level of superior
colliculus in midbrain

Lateral geniculate nucleus

Edinger–Westphal nucleus

Ciliary ganglion

Short ciliary nerves

Torch

Figure 2

Pathways for light reflex. Light in one eye causes
direct and consensual constriction of the pupil.

NYSTAGMUS

This often causes confusion but in practice there are only a few possible causes. Do not worry about a few jerks at the extremes of eye movement (**physiological gaze-evoked nystagmus**) – this is normal. Nystagmus nearly always implies **ear** or **posterior fossa** disease.

Nystagmus to one side with greater amplitude in the ipsilateral eye (eg nystagmus on looking right, which is most marked in the right eye) is caused by:

> **Ipsilateral cerebellar/brainstem** lesion
> Vascular/neoplastic (primary/secondary)/demyelinating/ infective
> **Contralateral vestibular** lesion (fast to contralateral side)
> **Peripheral**
>> Fatigable/seen on positional testing
>> Cochlear dysfunction   Labyrinthitis
>>> Ménière's disease
>>> Head injury
>>> BPPV (see Comment)
>>> Nerve VIII disease   Acoustic neuroma
>>> Viral neuronitis (acute vertigo/nystagmus)
> **Central**
>> Not fatigable/present at rest
>> Vestibular nuclear damage   Vascular
>>> Neoplastic
>>> Demyelinating
>>> Drugs (phenytoin/carbamazepine)

Vertical nystagmus implies central brainstem pathology:

> **Upgaze**   Level of superior colliculus
> **Downgaze**   Level of foramen magnum

COMMENT

Benign paroxysmal positional vertigo (BPPV), due to dislodged otoliths in the semilunar canals, presents with vertigo and nystagmus on movement. Treatment is symptomatic, and repositioning the otoliths (eg Epley's manoeuvre).

CASE 116

INTERNUCLEAR OPHTHALMOPLEGIA

This is a favourite short case. Invariably the patient will have MS and the other eye signs may reflect this.

Introduce and expose

Observe Multiple sclerosis (case 93 – young/ataxic speech/wheelchair)

Acuity Normal

Fields Normal

Pupils May have relative afferent pupillary defect (Marcus–Gunn pupil, impaired direct but preserved consensual light reflex) due to previous optic/retrobulbar neuritis

Movements

Decreased adduction/lag in adducting eye

Nystagmus (fast phase outwards) in abducting eye

Fundi May have optic atrophy (case 125)

COMMENT

Causes Bilateral   Demyelination (almost always)

Unilateral   Demyelination

Vascular (brainstem lesion ipsilateral to adducting eye)

The anatomical lesion is in the medial longitudinal fasciculus ipsilateral to the adducting eye (pathway connecting ipsilateral nerve VI nucleus to contralateral nerve III nucleus to allow conjugate gaze). In many cases bilateral damage has occurred.

NERVE III LESION

Oculomotor nerve palsy is sometimes called 'the tramp's pupil' because the eye looks **down and out**.

Introduce and expose

Observe Ptosis (complete/partial)
Eye looks out (may need to lift eyelid)

Acuity Normal

Fields Normal but limited by ptosis

Pupils Dilated (usually unreactive) if complete
Spared if partial

Movements

Nerve VI working so eye moves laterally
Nerve IV working so eye intorts on trying to look down and in
No other movements if complete
Variable movement during recovery

Fundi Normal/papilloedema if space-occupying lesion

Causes

Complete (motor to muscles and parasympathetic to pupil) –
sometimes called 'surgical' lesions and often painful
Aneurysm (ipsilateral posterior communicating artery)
Tumour

Incomplete (pupil spared and ptosis partial)

Nerve trunk infarction   Diabetes
Midbrain lesion   Vascular/demyelination
There are many other small-print causes including encephalitis and parasellar or sphenoidal wing meningiomas.

COMMENT

Investigation would include blood glucose, CT or MRI of the brain and carotid arteriography.

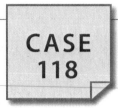

CASE 118   PTOSIS

Introduce and expose

Observe   Drooping of the eyelid
Upper part of the iris and pupil covered

The remainder of the examination is focused on defining a **cause**:

Observe   Bilateral ptosis (myasthenia/myotonia most likely)
Young females (idiopathic)

Acuity   Usually normal
Decreased with cataracts (myotonic dystrophy – case 98)

Fields   Normal

Pupils   **Small** but reactive (Horner's syndrome – case 112)
Dilated (nerve III palsy – case 117)
Otherwise normal

Movements
Decreased/'down and out' (nerve III palsy – case 117)
Fatigable/multiple muscles (myasthenia – case 99)
Otherwise normal

Fundi   **No red reflex** with cataracts (myotonic dystrophy)
Retinitis pigmentosa (case 127) with some mitochondrial
diseases

Extras   Variable (complex) neurological/myopathic problems with
mitochondrial diseases (rare)

COMMENT

The eyelid is kept up by the levator palpebrae superioris, which is innervated by the oculomotor (nerve III) nerve (small superior division), and by the muscle of Müller supplied by the sympathetic fibres (carried along the intracranial blood vessels). There will often be overactivity of the ipsilateral frontalis muscle making the forehead look more wrinkled on that side – if you are not careful you may misdiagnose a contralateral facial nerve (VII) palsy.

ABDUCENS NERVE (VI) PALSY

The abducens nerve (VI) can be injured anywhere along its course – commonly by vasculopathy of the vaso nervorum (mononeuritis multiplex, eg diabetes/sarcoid/vasculitis) or extrinsic compression.

Introduce and expose

Observe Normal

Acuity Normal

Fields Normal

Pupils Normal

Movements

Divergent squint at rest

No abduction/reduced abduction beyond the midline

Diplopia, worse when looking to the side of the lesion

Causes **Mononeuritis:** diabetes (case 53)/sarcoid (case 30)/rheumatoid (case 63)/SLE (case 64)/vasculitis

Raised ICP

Brainstem vascular disease

MS (case 93 – UMN, plaque in pons, ? associated with nerve VII palsy)

Beware myasthenia gravis (case 99) if not typical

Look for fatigability/worsening of diplopia with prolonged lateral gaze

THYROID EYE DISEASE

Remember that exophthalmos is caused by involvement of the extraocular muscles in Graves' disease (case 55).

Introduce and expose

Observe Exophthalmos/lid lag/chemosis

Acuity Normal (decreased if optic nerve compression)

Fields Normal (enlarged blind spot if papilloedema)

Pupils Normal

Movements

Decreased movement not confined to any single cranial nerve lesion

Superior and medial recti are often the most affected causing variable diplopia (mimicking nerve III lesion)

Fundi Usually normal/papilloedema if excessive inflammation of orbital muscles

Optic atrophy if this is prolonged

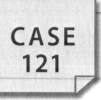

STRABISMUS

Congenital squint (strabismus) should be distinguished from other eye movement disorders and causes of diplopia.

The angle between the axis of the two eyes does not change with eye movement

There is no diplopia

There may be decreased acuity in the non-fixing eye

When assessing a squint you should perform the cover/uncover test.

Ask the patient to fix vision on your finger held at arm's length from the patient's face

Cover the deviated eye then the other in turn

The axis of the deviated eye will move from its position when the good eye is covered, and return to position when re-covered.

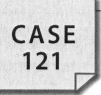

FUNDOSCOPY

Fundoscopy, or direct ophthalmoscopy, requires practice to look slick during the examination and to obtain good views of the retina. The pupils should be dilated, or fundoscopy assessed on a model.

Introduce and expose Sit the patient in a chair looking forwards. Warn the patient that you will be shining a bright light into the eye, and that you will be very close to the face.

Assemble the equipment and ensure that the ophthalmoscope is set to produce the largest plain white light with the dioptre setting at '0'.

Examine the external eye briefly if time allows (acuity, visual fields, pupils, eye movements).

If the patient is wearing glasses, ask for them to be removed. Turn off the lights in the room.

Use your **right** eye to examine the patient's **right** eye.

Looking through the ophthalmoscope, point the light at the pupil. You should see the **red reflex** (back of the retina) – if this is absent the patient may have a cataract.

Move in towards the patient's eye, tracking the red reflex. You may place your hand on the patient's forehead to prevent you from bumping into him or her. The thumb can be used to raise the upper eyelid gently to prevent blinking.

Find a blood vessel. Use the dioptre dial to **focus** the image. Track the blood vessel back to the optic disc.

From the **disc**, inspect the **four quadrants** (nasal/temporal, upper/lower). Inspect the **macula** (free of blood vessels, lateral to the disc).

Ask the patient to look briefly into the light – examine the **fovea**.

Repeat with your **left** eye to examine the patient's **left** eye. Thank the patient, ensure that he or she is comfortable and turn on the lights.

DIABETIC EYE DISEASE

This is one of the most common short cases in any exam. You should be absolutely sure what you may see and how to present it. There is no substitute for examining the eyes of patients with diabetes – do not rely on picture books alone.

Introduce and expose

Observe BM fingerprick testing marks on fingers (look when shaking hands)

Acuity May be decreased (cataracts/maculopathy)

Fields Normal/central scotoma if macular damage

Movements
Normal/nerve VI or partial nerve III lesions (mononeuritis)

Fundi **Background**
Microaneurysms
Dot/blot haemorrhages
Hard exudates
Pre-proliferative as above with:
Flame haemorrhages
Soft exudates
Proliferative as above with:
Neovascularisation (new, often disorganised vessels especially at the disc/macula)
Risk of vitreous haemorrhage/retinal detachment/ glaucoma
Treated
Photocoagulation scars:
Recent = pale
Old = pigmented
Maculopathy
Any stage of retinopathy at the macula – more risk to vision

COMMENT

Treated proliferative retinopathy is commonly seen in exams as the signs are stable and usually 'barn door'. After you have finished examining the fundus try to be bold with your presentation: 'This patient has treated proliferative diabetic retinopathy as evidenced by the haemorrhages, exudates and laser photocoagulation scars. I would like to examine him or her for further complications of diabetes and check his or her blood glucose.'

CASE 124

HYPERTENSIVE EYE DISEASE

Introduce and expose

Observe

Acuity   Usually normal

Fields   Normal/enlarged blind spot if papilloedema

Pupils

Movements

Fundi   Grade I   Arteriolar narrowing
                         'Silver wiring'
          Grade II   + 'AV nipping' – narrowing of the vessels
                         where veins and arterioles cross
          Grade III   + flame haemorrhages/'cotton-wool' spots
                         (exudates)
          Grade IV   + papilloedema

COMMENT

Grade III or IV implies accelerated hypertension. Grade III is easy to confuse with pre-proliferative diabetic retinopathy, but there are usually fewer microaneurysms/haemorrhages (dot/blot). If in doubt, confess your ignorance and suggest that you check the blood pressure and the blood glucose.

CASE 125

OPTIC ATROPHY

Introduce and expose

Observe MS (case 93 – young/ataxic speech/wheelchair)

Acuity Decreased

Fields **Central scotoma** (case 110)/bitemporal hemianopia (case 109) if chiasmatic compression

Pupils Normal at rest
Relative afferent pupillary defect (Marcus–Gunn pupil, impaired direct but preserved consensual light reflex)

Movements
Normal

Fundi Pale optic discs
Pathological cupping in glaucoma

Causes

Primary Damage to nerve
Optic neuritis – MS (case 93)
Compression (glaucoma/tumour/Paget's disease (case 70)/ thyroid eye disease (case 102))
Ischaemic
Toxic (methanol/lead/quinine)
Infective (syphilis)
Nutritional (vitamin B_{12} deficiency)
Hereditary (Friedreich's ataxia (case 103)/Leber's optic atrophy)

Secondary
To chronic papilloedema (case 126)

Consecutive
To retinal disease:
Retinitis pigmentosa (case 127)
Choroiditis

PAPILLOEDEMA

Introduce and expose

Observe

Acuity Usually normal (may be decreased)

Fields **Increased size of blind spot**
Concentric constriction if severe (case 111)

Pupils Depends on pathology

Movement
Depends on pathology

Fundi Loss of venous pulsation (early)
Blurred disc margin
Swelling of optic nerve head:
Localised haemorrhages
Other signs of hypertensive retinopathy (case 124)

Extras Signs/symptoms of raised intracranial pressure (case 95)

Causes **Intracranial space-occupying lesion:**
Tumour
Abscess
Haematoma
Accelerated hypertension
Idiopathic intracranial hypertension
Hydrocephalus
Hypercapnia
Central retinal vein thrombosis
Thyroid eye disease (case 120)
Hypocalcaemia
Severe anaemia
Guillain–Barré syndrome (raised CSF protein)

RETINAL PIGMENTATION

Introduce and expose

Observe   Complex syndromes with retinitis pigmentosa (may be with a hearing aid (Usher's syndrome))

Acuity   May be decreased depending on the amount of macular damage

Fields   Variable/possible central scotoma (case 110)
May have concentric constriction (case 111)

Pupils   Normal

Movements
Ophthalmoplegia with some mitochondrial myopathies (eg Kearns–Sayre syndrome – rare!)

Fundi   Variable pigmentary changes depending on the cause

Extras   Signs of diabetes (old laser photocoagulation scars)

Causes
Race   Dark skin/pigmented retina
Senile degeneration
Especially macular
Retinitis pigmentosa
Peripheries first → widespread
Night blindness → tunnel vision → generalised poor acuity
Often inherited, many genetic/mitochondrial syndromes
Old choroiditis
'Lumps of coal' lesions in isolated areas
Laser photocoagulation
Treated diabetic proliferative retinopathy (old)

CASE 128

FACIAL NERVE (VII) PALSY

Unable to:

Close eye(s) (eyeball rolls up – Bell's phenomenon)
Raise eyebrow(s) (spared in unilateral UMN lesions)
Blow out cheeks/whistle
Show teeth

Although the nerve VII supplies the anterior two-thirds of taste, patients rarely notice/complain of taste sensation changes.

Unilateral facial nerve palsies are divided into complete (LMN) or incomplete (UMN).

LMN
All muscles of facial expression weak
Nerve damaged between the nucleus (brainstem) and the face
By observing whether there is hyperacusis (sensitivity to loud noises – nerve to stapedius) or loss of taste (chorda tympani), you can say whether the lesion is above or below the facial canal (both preserved if below)

Causes
Bell's palsy (idiopathic)
Ramsay–Hunt syndrome (herpes zoster at the external auditory meatus/soft palate)
Cerebellopontine angle tumour (case 130)
Mononeuritis (case 119 – especially sarcoid/diabetes)
Parotid tumour/middle-ear disease/pontine lesions
Vascular/demyelinating

UMN
The UMN fibres are damaged between the cortex and nucleus. As there is input from both hemispheres to the upper facial muscles a lesion of one cortex or its tracts will not cause weakness of the forehead. UMN lesions spare the upper face

Causes
Cerebrovascular accident (case 92)

Bilateral The differential diagnosis is different as all the causes listed already are rare bilaterally

Causes

Nuclear	Vascular/demyelinating
Infranuclear	Guillain–Barré syndrome/sarcoidosis (case 30)
Muscular	Myasthenia gravis (case 99)/myotonia (case 98)

CAVERNOUS SINUS SYNDROME

Clinical findings

Nerves III, IV, VI	Subtotal/total ophthalmoplegia (pain)	
Nerve V	Ophthalmic	Loss of sensation in V1 territory
	Loss of corneal reflex (afferent)	
	Maxillary	Variably involved
Causes	Thrombosis in the cavernous sinus	
	Tumour (meningioma, pituitary tumours, craniopharyngiomas)	

The cavernous sinus lies laterally to the sella turcica, and receives the venous drainage from the ophthalmic veins and, indirectly, the face. Infection entering the facial veins (eg after trauma) can cause a thrombosis of the sinus and compression of the many nerves passing through it.

CASE 130

CEREBELLO-PONTINE ANGLE LESION

Clinical findings

Nerve V	Ophthalmic Loss of corneal reflex
	Maxillary
	Mandibular Mild weakness of muscles of mastication
Nerve VI	Ipsilateral lateral rectus palsy
Nerve VII	LMN facial weakness (case 128)
	Loss of anterior two-thirds of taste/hyperacusis
Nerve VIII	Sensorineural deafness

Cerebellar signs

For example, nystagmus (if large tumour)

Causes   Tumours   Acoustic neuroma/meningioma
(others rarely)

The cerebellopontine angle is a small triangular fossa between the cerebellum, pons and petrous temporal bone from nerve V to cranial nerve IX.

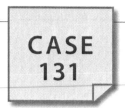

CASE 131

JUGULAR FORAMEN SYNDROME

Clinical findings

Nerves IX/X	Decreased palatal movement
	Loss of gag reflex
Nerve XI	Wasting of sternocleidomastoid
	Weak head turn to contralateral side
	Weak shoulder shrug (upper part of trapezius)

Causes   Tumour

Glomus jugulare tumour (blue eardrum, pulse audible to patient due to AV anastomosis in tumour)

Base-of-skull fracture

Paget's disease (case 70)

Jugular venous thrombosis

BULBAR PALSY

It is difficult to tell these two apart just by listening. The associated features (LMN = bulbar, UMN = pseudobulbar) are better indicators.

Nerves IX/X	Poor palatal movement/loss of gag reflex
Nerve XII	Weak/wasted tongue/fasciculation
Speech	Poor quality/as if nose blocked due to no movement of the soft palate
Cough	Poor cough impulse (may be very feeble)
	Nasal regurgitation on swallowing
	May have NG tube or feeding gastrostomy
Causes	MND (case 97)
	Syringobulbia (case 100)
	Guillain–Barré syndrome
	Medullary lesions (vascular/demyelinating/tumour)
	Myasthenia gravis (case 99) may produce a similar picture, but it is not truly a bulbar palsy

PSEUDOBULBAR PALSY

Clinical findings

Spastic tongue (small/decreased/slow movement/no fasciculation)

Poor palatal movement/gag reflex unreliable

'Donald Duck' speech

Extras   Jaw jerk brisk (usually)

UMN signs in limbs

Emotionally labile

Causes   Bilateral CVA (case 92) – internal capsule

Demyelination

MND (case 97): UMN/LMN signs in limbs/cranial nerves **without sensory signs**

Degenerative cerebral disease

THE 3 Ds

'Ask this patient some questions.'

This is not the same as asking you to take a history but has the specific aim of directing you to find out whether there is **dysarthria, dysphasia** or **dementia** (the 3 Ds).

You must establish handedness at some stage – this is better left until the end but should never be forgotten.

Introduce and expose

Observe   Evidence of hemiparesis (CVA – case 92)

Ask   'Please would you tell me your name and where you are.'
If there is obvious **dysarthria** go on to define it:

>**Bulbar** (case 132) – wasted tongue
>**Pseudobulbar** (case 133) – brisk jaw jerk
>**Cerebellar** (case 107) – nystagmus/ataxia

If there is no dysarthria or an inappropriate or incomplete answer test for **dysphasia**:

Receptive (sensory)

>'Please touch your nose'/'Stick out your tongue'
>'Touch your right ear with your left hand'
>Speech often fluent but low content

If there is no response or a completely inappropriate response you will be unable to proceed. Tell the examiner 'This patient has a marked receptive dysphasia (with/without preserved speech). This would indicate a lesion in Wernicke's area (with/without involvement of Broca's area). The most likely cause is a CVA. I would like to look for predisposing factors (HTN/AF/ bruits, etc)'.

If there is no receptive dysphasia, test for expressive dysphasia:

Expressive (motor)

      'Would you tell me what this is?'

      Show the patient a watch/pen/torch, etc.

      Ask the patient what the hands/lid/bulb, etc are

If there is a problem this would suggest a lesion of Broca's area. If there is no significant problem go on to quickly test higher cerebral function (see p. 5). If everything was normal you missed something!

VIVA QUESTIONS

What is being done to encourage early diagnosis and prevention of stroke?

Public health campaigns are aimed at encouraging patients with suspected stroke to present to hospital early. The Act FAST campaign uses new facial droop, arm weakness and speech difficulty as markers of potential stroke requiring urgent medical assessment.

In hospital, healthcare professionals are encouraged to use the **recognition of stroke in the emergency room** (ROSIER) score:

Loss of consciousness or syncope/seizure activity	−1 each
Asymmetrical weakness of face/arm/leg	+1 each
Speech disturbance/visual field defect	+1 each

Total score is between −2 and +5. Scores 0 make acute CVA likely.

If a patient's neurological signs have resolved by the time that he or she is assessed, ROSIER cannot be used. The ABCD^2 score is used to risk stratify suspected TIAs to guide further investigations and treatment:

Age	>60 years	1 point
Blood pressure	>140/90 mmHg	1 point
Clinical features	Asymmetrical weakness	2 points
	Speech disturbance	1 point
Duration	>60 min	2 points
	10–60 min	1 point
Diabetes	If present	1 point

A score of 6+ gives an 8% chance of stroke within 48 h. High-risk patients are those with a score of 4 or more, or patients with two or more TIAs in a week (crescendo TIAs), and should be given aspirin 300 mg daily, with specialist investigation within 24 h.

What is the differential diagnosis of a patient presenting with spastic paraparesis?

The term 'spastic paraparesis' refers to pyramidal weakness of both legs and indicates a lesion in either the thoracic or the cervical spinal cord. The most important cause to exclude is spinal cord compression, because this may require prompt neurosurgical intervention.

The most common cause in a young patient is MS. In elderly people the most common cause is cervical spondylosis. Other causes include hereditary spastic paraparesis, parasagittal lesions, syringomyelia and subacute combined degeneration of the cord.

What causes of papilloedema do you know?

By definition, papilloedema means optic disc swelling secondary to raised ICP – the causes are therefore those of raised ICP, and include mass lesions (tumour/haematoma), diffuse inflammation (encephalitis), processes that interfere with CSF reabsorption (hydrocephalus/cerebral venous thrombosis) and idiopathic (benign) intracranial hypertension.

Optic disc swelling secondary to inflammation/infiltration is termed 'papillitis', and is more often unilateral, and usually leads to significant visual impairment.

What is the law on driving after a first fit?

The patient will not be allowed to drive for a period of 6 months from the date of the seizure (5 years for LGV/PCV drivers) and must remain seizure free before a licence is returned. The DVLA must be informed.

Patients with established epilepsy must be fit free for 1 year or only have seizures while asleep for 3 years. LGV/PCV drivers must be free of seizures and off medication for 10 years before they may reapply for a licence.

Special consideration may be given when the seizure is clearly associated with a non-recurring provoking cause, eg eclamptic seizure.

PSYCHIATRY

Examination of the mental state

There is no fundamental difference between the approach to a psychiatric long case and the approach to any other medical case. The length and detail of the history are greater and the Mental State Examination (MSE) takes over from the physical examination in importance. You must be sure, however, to exclude organic disease that may lead to psychiatric disturbance, eg SLE (psychosis)/thyroid disease (depression), and look for the physical complications of psychiatric disease, eg chronic liver disease (alcoholism), or treatments, eg movement disorders (psychotropic medication).

Your overall aim is to produce a formulation that includes the differential diagnosis and the aetiology:

Differential diagnosis
>**Organic psychoses**
>**Functional psychoses**
>**Non-psychotic disorders**
>**Personality disorders**

The aetiology
>**Predisposing factors**
>**Precipitating factors**
>**Maintaining factors**

You should also be able to comment on appropriate investigations, treatments and the prognosis.

Introduce yourself and establish a rapport. This may be part of the observed examination, and you will be marked on your ability to establish rapport, and on your questioning style and ability to define the problem. It is hard to be relaxed under scrutiny, but telling the patient that you are nervous because of the importance of the exam and that you feel as if you are taking your driving test again may break the ice!

On starting questioning **make good eye contact**. Start with **open questions** such as 'Would you please tell me what has been going on in your life recently'. Try not to interrupt the patient, give him or her time to speak. Use **active listening** (nodding, vocal prompts such as 'Go on'). Use **closed questions** to define more detailed points.

PC	In detail, using the patient's own words
HPC	Describe the development of symptoms
	Ask about any associated symptoms
	Duration/timing of illness (relapses, remissions)
	How was it diagnosed?
PMH	Including past psychiatric history
	Note any previous episodes of the same or similar symptoms as the presenting complaint (you may be the first to recognise a crisis in the patient's past that may have been psychotic or depressive)
FH	Commonly positive for psychiatric disease
SH	Personal:
	Childhood/school
	Sexual development/relationships
	Marriage/children
	Occupation (past and present)/job problems
	Forensic (trouble with the police/convictions)
	Pre-morbid personality
	Interests/relations with others
	Previous level of function
	Coping skills/resources
	Social history as with any medical history
	Smoking, alcohol, drugs (prescribed and recreational)
DH	Antidepressants/psychotropics
	Over the counter/alternative remedies
ROS	Especially somatic symptoms of psychiatric disease:
	Appetite changes/weight loss
	Sleep disturbance/loss of libido
	Lack of energy/motivation
	Symptoms underlying psychiatric disorder:
	Chronic disease (eg chronic pain)

Mental State Examination

Behaviour/Appearance
Dress/self-care/eye contact/rapport
Conscious level/posture/involuntary movements

Speech Speed/quantity/quality (subject matter/clarity)

Mood Subjective/objective
Variability/lability
Autonomic activity (sweaty, etc)

Thought (form/content)
Abnormal beliefs/preoccupations/suicidality (case 136)

Perception
Illusions/hallucinations/passivity
Depersonalisation/derealisation

Orientation
Time/place/person

Attention/concentration
Months/days backwards or serial 7s

Memory Short term: address/digit span
Long term: Prime Minister/famous dates/past life

Abstraction
What is the difference between a dwarf and a child?
Test meanings of proverbs/sayings

Insight Does he or she realise that he or she is ill?
Is he or she willing to be treated?

General examination
All systems as with any medical examination

Investigations
Psychosocial (including collateral history)
Medical (for underlying organic disease/complications)

Treatments
Psychological
Physical/medical

DEPRESSION

The patient is likely to know that he or she has this diagnosis, and with luck the patient or the examiner will tell you at the start.

PC		Find out what the first symptoms were/when they happened
HPC	**Emotional**	Sad/helpless/anxious/agitated
	Cognitive	Self-dislike/blame
		Worthlessness/hopelessness/suicidality
		Poor thinking/indecisiveness
	Biological	Sleep (poor with early morning waking)
		Appetite/weight (usually down, may be up)
		Libido/energy/concentration (all decreased)
		Diurnal variation (worse in the morning)
		New symptoms (headache/pains/dizziness...)
	Precipitants	Losses (bereavement/job/divorce/health)
		Life events (usually stressful)
PMH		Depressive/manic/psychotic episodes
		Serious/chronic medical illness
FH		Bipolar affective disorder
		Family member with serious illness (eg son with leukaemia)
SH	**Personal**	Childhood losses/insecurity/abuse
		Relationships/marriage/divorce/separation
		Occupation/stress at work/unemployment
		Money problems/housing problems
		Friends/interests
	Pre-morbid	Low self-esteem
		Level of function/coping skills
		Locus of control
		Smoking/alcohol (may be excessive)/drugs
DH		Treatments
		Predisposing, eg β-blockers, steroids, antiarrhythmics

ROS   Thyroid/other general disorders

Mental State Examination

Behaviour	Poor eye contact/posture/self-neglect
	Increased or decreased activity
Speech	Slow/little spontaneous/coherent
Mood	Low
Thought	Worthless/hopeless/guilt/blame/suicide
Perception	May have hallucinations/nihilistic delusions
Orientation	Usually normal
Attention	May be poor
Memory	Impaired if attention decreased
Insight	Often preserved

EXAMINATION

General appearance

Look for signs of general medical illness

INVESTIGATIONS

Exclude organic disease

FBC/U&Es/CRP/calcium/TFTs

ECG if palpitations

TREATMENT

If suicidal (case 136) may need to 'section' under the Mental Health Act

Psychological	For mild–moderate depression
	Consider CBT (guided/computerised)
	Physical activity (especially structure group activity)
Pharmacological	For moderate–severe depression/persistent symptoms despite psychological interventions
Electroconvulsive	For severe/psychotic depression

Inpatient admission

Selective serotonin reuptake inhibitors (SSRIs)

    Fluoxetine/paroxetine/citalopram/sertraline

        Risk of upper GI bleeding/hyponatraemia

Tricyclic antidepressants (TCAs)

    Amitriptyline/imipramine/clomipramine

        Antimuscarinic side-effects/dangerous in overdose

Monoamine oxidase inhibitors (MAOIs)

    Phenelzine (irreversible)/moclobemide (reversible)

        Avoid tyramine-rich foods (cheese, yeast extract, tofu)

Other agents

    Mirtazapine/venlafaxine/reboxetine

        May be preferred if multiple co-morbidities/drug interactions

Antidepressant efficacy should be assessed 2–4 weeks after starting treatment.

Patients may be using over-the-counter St John's wort, a herbal remedy. This can be effective for mild depression, but is a potent enzyme inducer and can affect many other drug levels. It should not be taken with other antidepressants.

COMMENT

Often patients with anxiety disorders develop depression and features of both conditions may coexist ('anxious depression'). During the history you should look for symptoms for anxiety:

Palpitations	Tachycardia	Bowel disturbance
Sweating	Irritability	Swallowing problems
Phobias	Panic attacks	Agoraphobia
Dizziness	Pins and needles	

Be sure to elucidate any thyroid or cardiac disease and check whether the patient is using β-agonist inhalers.

ASSESSING SUICIDALITY

You may be asked to assess a patient's risk of suicide. The key is taking a good history.

Introduce yourself and establish rapport

Suicidal intent	Do they have any thoughts of ending their life?
	Are these active (killing themselves) or passive (wanting to die)?
	How often do they have these thoughts?
	How persistent are these thoughts?
	Are they able to control these thoughts?
Motivation	To die/to punish self/others
	Recent loss of significant other?
	View of death (eg reunite with loved one)
	Reasons for living
Past behaviour	Any previous suicide/self-harm attempts
	Alcohol/drug use
	Panic attacks/anxiety
	Recent life stressors/crises
Current state	Affect (depressed/psychotic)
	Anhedonia/hopelessness
	Intoxicated
	Energy/motivation levels
	Physical/chronic Illness
	Do they still want to kill themselves now?
Suicide plan	How? Is the equipment available? Likely to succeed?
	Where? When? Expectation of discovery?
	Preparation? Rehearsal?
	Did they leave a note/plans for after death?

There is no 'golden rule'. The balance is between overdiagnosing (risk of depriving patient of liberty) and underdiagnosing (risk of suicide).

PSYCHOSIS/ SCHIZOPHRENIA

PC   'What has been going on in your life recently?'

HPC   Prodrome   Loss of interest/poor hygiene

                               Change in mood/decline in function

             Diagnostic features of schizophrenia (see Comment)

             Exclude mania/depression/intoxication/organic brain disorders, eg epilepsy

             Look for precipitating factors/recent life events

PMH   Previous episodes of psychiatric disease (especially psychotic)

             Sensory impairment (deaf/blind) in elderly people

FH   Positive family history is common

SH   **Personal**   Birth trauma

                               Erratic school performance (especially boys)

                               Unable to have a long-term relationship

                               Poor employment/criminal record

                               Low income, difficult social circumstances

                               Poor housing/living rough

             Pre-morbid   Schizoaffective/schizotypal personality

                               Withdrawn/eccentric/paranoid

             Smoking/alcohol (especially excessive)/drugs

DH   Treatment, eg depot injections

             Precipitants, eg steroids

             Illicit drugs (cannabis, amphetamines) as precipitants

ROS   Epilepsy/headaches (brain tumour)

             Alcohol withdrawal

Mental State Examination

Behaviour   Self-neglect/abnormal movements (treatment effect)

Speech	Varied/incomprehensible
	Neologisms/'clangs' (rhyming associations)
Mood	Blunted/inappropriate affect (laughing, etc)
Thought	Insertion/withdrawal/broadcasting
	Abnormal beliefs (eg that they are Jesus)
	Direct communication with media, eg TV
Perception	Auditory hallucinations (third person/thought echo/
	running commentary)
	Passivity feelings
Orientation	Person (eg Jesus Christ/being talked to by TV)
	Often normal
Attention	Often poor
Memory	Decreased if attention poor
Insight	Often poor; depends on degree of treatment

Note that some forms of schizophrenia have more negative features (poverty of speech/movement/motivation, blunted affect, etc).

EXAMINATION

General appearance

Signs of drug use/brain tumour

INVESTIGATIONS

Psychosocial investigations

Drug screen/EEG /CT scan

TREATMENT

Supportive   Decrease stress in the environment

Decrease expressed emotion in the family

Rehabilitation, eg day centres

Drugs

Acute	Atypical antipsychotics (eg olanzapine/risperidone)
	Neuroleptics (eg haloperidol/ chlorpromazine/sulpiride)
Chronic	Oral/depot, eg flupentixol

COMMENT

The diagnosis of schizophrenia is indicated by one or more of the following symptoms:

Disorders of:

    Thought possession

    Thought insertion

    Thought withdrawal

    Thought broadcasting

Auditory hallucinations of:

    The patient's own thoughts out loud (thought echo)

    People discussing the patient in the third person

    Voices forming a running commentary

Passivity:

    Feeling under control of an outside influence

Delusions:

    Persistent beliefs (culturally/physically impossible)

    Delusional perception

Or two or more of the following:

    Persistent hallucinations

    Incoherent/irrelevant speech/mannerisms

    Neologisms

    Catatonic phenomena

    Negative symptoms

EATING DISORDERS

Anorexia nervosa is characterised by a morbid fear of fatness and distortion of body image with a refusal to maintain a healthy weight. Bulimia nervosa patients may have a low, normal or high body weight, but an inability to control eating behaviour with episodes of overeating (binges) followed by compensatory fasting/vomiting/exercise (purges).

PC   When was the condition first brought to medical attention? Why?

HPC   Body weight in the past (fat/thin)
How the patient has dieted/controlled calories
Eating behaviour – binge episodes
Exercise/purging behaviour
Ask about body image/fear of fatness
Menstrual history/amenorrhoea
Previous investigations for diarrhoea/metabolic diseases

PMH   Diabetes/thyroid disease

FH   Increased eating disorders in family members

SH   **Personal**
Disturbed family relations
Avoidance of maturity/sexual relationships
Denial of family problems
Parental discord (divorce/separation)
Smoking/alcohol/drugs (eg stimulants)

DH   Laxatives/diuretics

ROS   Raynaud's phenomenon/sensitivity to cold is common
Excess (lanugo) hair on face/back
Exclude endocrine/digestive disorders – diabetes/thyroid disease/inflammatory bowel disease/coeliac disease/ovarian/pituitary disease

Mental State Examination

Behaviour	Normal
Speech	Normal
Mood	Anxious/depressed
	Unconcerned about health
Thought	Concerned about/abnormal body image
	Assess any suicidality

Perception/orientation/attention/memory usually normal

Insight	Lacking regarding health

EXAMINATION

General appearance

Thin/cold peripheries/lanugo hair

Weight/height – calculate BMI (weight in kg/height in m^2)

Check for hyper-/hypothyroidism, etc.

Parotid hypertrophy/dental erosion with repeated vomiting

INVESTIGATIONS

Psychosocial – family relationships

Glucose/thyroid function tests

U&Es (low K$^+$ with purgatives/diuretics)

Low serum protein/FSH/LH

ACTH increased (stress response)

TREATMENT

Restore body weight

Behavioural programme

Psychotherapy (family/individual therapy)

May need to move away from family situation

May need antidepressant medication

SUBSTANCE ABUSE

This may relate to any drug but most often it applies to alcohol, in which case there may be an overlap with chronic liver disease. The patient develops a **compulsion** to use the drug, **increased tolerance** to its effects and **withdrawal symptoms** on stopping. You must look out for biological, psychological and social complications (eg liver disease, changes in mood and marriage breakdown) and salience or stereotypical behaviour.

PC　　When first brought to medical attention? Why?

HPC　　When did they first take the drug?
　　　　When did they begin to use it regularly/heavily?
　　　　Why did they first use the drug?
　　　　Peer pressure/anxiety/depression/availability
　　　　How do they obtain (and pay for) the drug?
　　　　How do they use it? (inject, smoke, etc)
　　　　How much do they use (eg units of alcohol)?
　　　　What effects did and does the drug have for them?
　　　　Any tolerance (do they need more for the same effect)?
　　　　Any withdrawal effects?
　　　　Fits/delerium tremens/cold turkey/anxiety
　　　　When did they first have problems with the drug? What?

PMH　　Depression/other psychiatric history
　　　　Chronic illness/chronic pain (eg opioids)

FH　　Increased addictive behaviour in family members

SH　　Childhood exposure to addictive behaviour
　　　　Abusive/neglected childhood
　　　　Poor performance at school/work
　　　　High-risk occupation (barman/sales rep/doctor)
　　　　Criminal record (especially drink-/drug-related crimes, how to pay for habit, eg theft, prostitution; violence)
　　　　Marital/relationship history (divorce/aggression)

Home/financial situation (money all spent on habit)

Alcohol, smoking and drug history (all relevant to any drug)

Alcohol Number of units per week/typical drinking day

Binges? Periods of abstinence?

CAGE questionnaire (2+ 'yes' = investigate further)

C Have you ever felt you ought to **c**ut down on your drinking?

A Have people **a**nnoyed you by criticising your drinking?

G Have you ever felt **g**uilty about drinking?

E Have you ever had a drink first thing in the morning to steady your nerves of get rid of a hangover (an **e**ye-opener)?

DH Prescribed/over-the-counter/illicit medications

ROS Identify associations with the specific drug, eg:

Alcohol   Cardiomyopathy/myopathy

Gastritis/oesophagitis/pancreatitis/hepatitis/chronic liver disease

Malnutrition

Cerebellar degeneration/stroke/falls/Wernicke–Korsakoff syndrome

Intravenous drugs

Hepatitis/HIV/endocarditis/infections

Mental State Examination

Behaviour	Poor self-care/abnormal movements/withdrawal
Speech	Cerebellar/slurred
Mood	Anxiety/depression
Thought	Preoccupation with drink/drugs/paranoia/suicide
Perception	
Orientation	Abnormal if intoxicated
Attention	Poor
Memory	Korsakoff's psychosis – retrograde and anterograde amnesia with confabulation
Insight?	'I can kick it'; but they haven't/can't

EXAMINATION

General appearance
>May be unkempt
>Signs of the complications of the substance used
>Needle marks/phlebitis/scars/abscesses

INVESTIGATIONS

>FBC, U&Es, LFTs, others depending on type of drug
>Hepatitis/HIV serology if injecting/high risk
>Social investigations – collateral histories

TREATMENT

Acute   Treatment of withdrawal:

Alcohol	Chlordiazepoxide regimen
	Vitamin supplementation® eg Pabrinex, thiamine, vitamin B
Opiates	Symptomatic/methadone

Treatment of overdose

>See (case 142)

Long term

Support	Family/social
	Alcoholics/narcotics anonymous
	Psychological/psychiatric services
Drugs	Antabuse/methadone

Treatment of any underlying mood disorder.

COMMENT

The drugs most often abused are: alcohol/opiates/hallucinogens/ amphetamines/cannabis/solvents. There may be a history of abuse of several drugs over the course of the illness (consecutively/concurrently), and each of these should be mentioned.

VIVA QUESTIONS

What medications may cause parkinsonism?

Parkinsonism refers to the combination of bradykinesia, extrapyramidal rigidity and tremor. Drug-induced parkinsonism is the most common cause after Parkinson's disease. The drugs most often implicated are the neuroleptics (major tranquillisers) such as haloperidol. Newer agents (atypical antipsychotics) are less likely to produce extrapyramidal side-effects. Their mode of action is primarily dopamine receptor blockade.

How would you assess whether someone was demented?

The term 'dementia' refers to a chronic, acquired cognitive impairment. Alzheimer's disease and progressive cerebrovascular disease (vascular dementia) are the most common causes. Typically the first symptom is memory impairment. Often the patient is less aware of the problem than the family. It is thus essential to take a detailed history from both patient and close family members. Neurological examination is typically normal. Neuropsychological examination is the key to diagnosis, most often administered in an abbreviated form, such as the Mini-Mental State Examination (MMSE). Depression can sometimes masquerade as dementia ('depressive pseudo-dementia'), and must be looked for carefully – it is readily treatable.

THERAPEUTICS

WRITING A DRUG CHART

The key points when writing a prescription are safety and clarity. Drug charts vary from hospital to hospital – you should be familiar with those in your medical school.

Patient identification

Ensure that the name, date of birth and hospital ID number are written clearly on the front of the chart and on any other pages where they are required.

Some charts have a space for the current ward, consultant team, date of admission, etc. If this information is expected then it should be provided.

Chart identification

Write Chart 1 of 1, Chart 1 of 2, etc in the appropriate space.

Allergies

Record any known or suspected allergies.

If known, describe the reaction, eg anaphylaxis, rash.

Drugs prescribed

Most charts have areas for once-only drugs, regular prescriptions inside, and as required (prn) drugs and some have a section for variable dose prescriptions, eg insulins.

Write the drug names clearly, in full, in capital letters.

Use approved generic names, except for drugs where the precise formulation matters (eg sustained-release diltiazem).

Write the dose clearly:

> Grams and milligrams can be abbreviated to g, mg
> Micro-/nanograms: units should be written in full
> Avoid unnecessary decimal points:
>> 3 mg not 3.0 mg
>> 500 mg not 0.5 g

For liquid preparations record the concentration and the delivered dose (weight preferred to volume):

> Drug: amoxicillin oral suspension 125 mg/5 ml
> Dose: 250 mg

State the route(s) of administration, eg po, iv/im

Note the times of day for the dose – for prn prescriptions, give a minimum dose interval, eg max every 4 hours.

Sign the prescription, write your name legibly next to your signature, and preferably your bleep number and designation.

Changing a dose or drug

It is good practice to completely rewrite any changes to a prescription, rather than altering an existing entry – this makes it easier when looking back to see what was changed and when.

Cross completely through the invalid entry, sign, name and date the change.

Controlled drug prescriptions

In hospital, controlled drugs such as morphine can be prescribed as any other drug. However, prescriptions for the patient to take home, on discharge or from clinic, have additional requirements.

The prescription must be indelibly written (printed prescriptions are allowed), be signed and dated, and give the prescriber's address (eg the address of the hospital/GP practice) and the patient's address. The total quantity to be supplied must be written in words and figures.

Example of dose and preparation:

> Oramorph concentrated oral solution 100 mg/5 ml
> Supply 120 ml (one hundred and twenty millilitres)
> 100 mg orally as required, maximum every 2 hours

REPORTING AN ADVERSE EVENT

Drug side-effects are monitored by the Medicines and Healthcare products Regulatory Agency (MHRA).

When to report side-effects

For established drugs, even well-recognised drug reactions should be reported if they are serious:

> Fatal/life-threatening events
>
> Events that result in disability/prolonged hospitalisation

Causality does not have to be proved – if you suspect a serious reaction may be caused by **any** drug, report it.

For newer drugs (marked with a black triangle symbol (▼) in the British National Formulary (BNF) **all** suspected reactions, however minor, should be reported. Any reaction that 'could conceivably be attributed' to a new drug should be reported, even if other drugs that may have been responsible were being given concurrently.

How to report side-effects

Use the Yellow Card Scheme:

> Yellow Cards are available at the back of the BNF or from your hospital pharmacy department
>
> Alternatively you can report using an online Yellow Card via the MHRA website (www.yellowcard.mhra.gov.uk)

Required information

The more information you are able to provide, the better, but do not be put off reporting a suspected reaction just because some details are unclear.

Patient details	Sex/age/weight/hospital ID number
Drug details	Drug name(s)/brand/batch number
	Dose/route of administration
	Date started/stopped/indication
Suspected reaction	Describe the reaction briefly
	Date reaction started/stopped
	Recovered/recovering/continuing
	Do you consider it to be serious?
Other drugs	Within the last 3 months (if known)
Medical history	

OVERDOSE

Accidental or deliberate poisoning with drugs is a common reason for presenting to the accident and emergency department (A&E). Common scenarios include: paracetamol, salicylates (ASA), opiates, benzodiazepines (BZD), tricyclic antidepressants (TCA), methanol/ethylene glycol (alcohols).

PC   Deliberate/accidental overdose
           What drug, when, how much, taken with anything else?

HPC   Any suicidal ideation?
           Nausea and vomiting are common
           Tinnitus/deafness with ASAs

SH   Alcohol history (regular drinking induces liver enzymes)

DH   Other medications

General appearance
           Appears intoxicated (alcohols, early)
           CNS agitation (ASA/TCA/alcohols later)
           CNS depression (opiates/BZDs/late presentation with any)
           Pupils pinpoint (opiates) or dilated (BZDs)

CVS   Bradycardia (β-blockers)
           Tachycardia/arrhythmias (ASA/TCA/alcohols)

Respiratory
           ↑ RR (compensating for acidosis – ASA, TCA, alcohols)
           ↓ RR (respiratory depression – opiates, BZDs)

Abdominal
           Jaundice (late presentation with paracetamol)

Investigations
           Drug levels, blood tests, ABG, ECG and monitoring

TREATMENT

Check with your local poisons unit or Toxbase online

If early presentation/slow release, ? activated charcoal/GI lavage

Supportive care, eg O_2, fluid resuscitation for hypotension/tachycardia, bicarbonate for acidosis, benzodiazepines for seizures

Specific antidotes:

Paracetamol	*N*-Acetylcysteine
Alcohols	Fomepizole or intravenous ethanol
Opiates	Naloxone
BZDs	Flumazenil (never in mixed overdose!)

Dialysis removes some drugs, eg lithium, ASA.

HUMAN IMMUNO-DEFICIENCY VIRUS

The number of people living with HIV infection, and the subsequent AIDS, is increasing worldwide.

HIV should be considered a chronic disease requiring long-term treatment and monitoring. The complications can affect any organ system. The patient may tell you that they are HIV positive, and may be well informed about their clinical history, viral load and treatment. Alternatively they may present with a history/signs suggesting underlying HIV infection/associated complication and there may be identifiable risk factors for HIV exposure.

Acute seroconversion illness
Occurs in up to 90%, but often not diagnosed.

A non-specific, transient, glandular fever-like illness at the time of antibody formation, within 3 months of HIV inoculation. Typical symptoms include fever, lymphadenopathy, maculopapular rash and flu-like and constitutional symptoms.

The acute phase usually lasts <2 weeks.

Common manifestations of HIV/AIDS
Careful examination including the skin, eyes and mucous membranes may reveal a number of the features below, and there may be a history of one or more of the specific organ system infections/malignancies.

General	Weight loss/anorexia/muscle wasting
	Lymphadenopathy/non-Hogkin's lymphoma
Skin	Seborrhoeic dermatitis
	Recurrent shingles (often different dermatomes)
	Molluscum contagiosum/intractable viral warts
	Kaposi's sarcoma
	Fungal nail infections
Mouth	Recurrent ulcers/candidiasis/URTI
	Oral hairy leukoplakia/chronic herpes simplex
Eyes	CMV retinitis

Respiratory

Recurrent bacterial pneumonia/fungal/TB

Pneumocystis jirovecii (*carinii*) pneumonia

GI Oesophageal candidiasis (odynophagia)

Cryptosporidiosis (chronic diarrhoea)

GU Chronic herpes simplex/anogenital warts

Invasive cervical carcinoma

Nephrotic syndrome (HIV-associated nephropathy)

Symptoms of concurrent sexually transmitted infections

CNS Cerebral toxoplasmosis/cryptococcal meningitis

Progressive multifocal leukoencephalopathy (PML)

HIV encephalopathy/AIDS–dementia complex

Modes of viral transmission

Unprotected sexual intercourse (most cases)

Intravenous drug needle sharing/needlestick injuries

Contaminated blood products/donor organs

Mother-to-child transmission in utero, peripartum or with breastfeeding

Treatment

Specific treatments for individual opportunistic infections/malignancies (eg co-trimoxazole for *Pneumocystis*, aciclovir for herpes viruses)

Highly active anti-retroviral therapy (HAART)

Treatment is aimed at reducing viral load and preventing progression to AIDS

Combination therapy with two nucleoside reverse transcriptase inhibitors + a non-nucleoside reverse transcriptase inhibitor or protease inhibitor

Issues

Treatment is not curative and must be continued lifelong – issues with compliance

Worldwide most of those infected have no access to treatment – sociopolitical ramifications

Stigma of diagnosis – cultural implications

EMERGENCY SKILLS

ASSESSMENT OF THE ACUTELY ILL PATIENT

Whenever you are presented with an unwell patient use a systematic approach to ensure that nothing is overlooked. Each stage should be assessed and any necessary treatment started before moving on to the next, ie do not move on to assessing breathing until you are happy that the airway is patent or a working airway adjunct is in place.

Airway

If the airway is not patent use an airway adjunct and seek early anaesthetic/critical care input

Give high-flow oxygen via a reservoir bag and mask

Breathing

Assess respiratory rate and chest movements

Check for tracheal deviation

Auscultate: is there equal air entry? Any crackles/wheeze?

If possible, sit the patient upright

Monitor O_2 saturations and adjust O_2 therapy accordingly

Circulation

Check pulse (large artery preferred – carotid/femoral)

Blood pressure – does the patient need fluid resuscitation?

Capillary refill time, peripheral pulses and temperature

Gain wide-bore intravenous access

Disability

Alert/responsive to **v**oice/**p**ain/**u**nresponsive (AVPU) or GCS (3/15 to 15/15, see Comment)

Pupil responses, limb movements

Blood sugar (see ABG opposite)

Exposure Temperature

Full systems examination

INVESTIGATIONS

Blood tests including coagulation screen, group and save

ECG, chest radiograph as soon as practical

The ABG is the most useful immediate investigation, giving:

PaO_2	**But** use SaO_2 to guide O_2 therapy
$PaCO_2$	CO_2 retaining? Hyperventilating?
pH	Acidotic? Renal failure, toxins, lactate
Lactate	Sign of tissue ischaemia, eg in sepsis
Glucose	Hypoglycaemia? Diabetic coma?

Potassium and other electrolytes, eg Na^+, Cl^-, Ca^{2+}

Haemoglobin

Treatment is supportive/resuscitative using an ABCDE approach and treatment for any identified/suspected underlying condition.

Common situations:

Severe sepsis (case 145)

Acute coronary syndrome (case 1)/cardiac arrest (case 21)

Acute pulmonary oedema (case 146)/severe asthma (case 147)

Upper GI bleed (case 39)

Acute kidney injury (case 41)/hyperkalaemia (case 148)

Diabetic ketoacidosis/hyperosmotic coma (case 53)

Thyroid storm (case 55)/myxoedema coma (case 56)

Addisonian crisis (case 58)

Cerebrovascular accident/subarachnoid haemorrhage (case 92)

Status epilepticus (case 94)

Acute poisoning, eg methanol/ethylene glycol (case 142)

Anaphylaxis (case 149)

COMMENT

The Glasgow Coma Scale assesses responsiveness on three axes. The minimum score for each is 1, so the minimum GCS is 3/15:

Eyes	Open spontaneously	4
	Open in response to voice	3
	Open in response to pain	2
	Unresponsive	1
Voice	Orientated and talking	5
	Confused	4
	Single words only	3
	Unintelligible noises	2
	No sounds	1
Movement	Obeys commands	6
	Localises to pain	5
	Withdraws from pain	4
	Abnormal flexion (decorticate)	3
	Abnormal extension (decerebrate)	2
	No movement	1

Record the total score and the axes, eg GCS 8/15 (E2, V2, M4).

SEVERE SEPSIS

Severe infection of any source must be treated promptly to prevent overwhelming sepsis with multiorgan failure and death.

ABCDE approach

Signs of septic source

Commonly chest/urinary infection; also abdominal/CNS

Look for cellulitis/necrotising fasciitis

Signs of severity

Tachycardia/arrhythmias

Tachypnoea (not exclusive to respiratory infections)

Temperature (hyperthermia/hypothermia)

Signs and symptoms of organ impairment

Acute confusion

Low BP (systolic <90 or ≤40 mmHg below patient's norm)

Reduced urine output

Immediate investigations as part of ABCDE

Bloods, ABG, ECG, chest radiograph – **do not delay treatment**

Specific investigations to identify organism

Blood cultures **before administering antibiotics**

Sputum, urine cultures, skin swabs if available

Immediate management as part of ABCDE

Fluid resuscitation if hypotension/lactate >4 mmol/l

Vasopressors (critical care input) if low BP despite fluid

Consider central venous pressure monitoring and ICU

Specific management for sepsis

Broad-spectrum antibiotics within 1 hour of admission

The systemic inflammatory response syndrome (SIRS) is present if there are two or more of:

Temperature <36.0 or >38.0°C

Tachycardia >90 beats/min

Tachypnoea >20/hypocapnia $PaCO_2$ <4.5 kPa

WBC <4 x 10^9/l or >12 × 10^9/l

SIRS + evidence of bacterial infection is sepsis. Severe sepsis is sepsis with organ dysfunction (eg shock, renal failure).

ACUTE PULMONARY OEDEMA

Sudden-onset pulmonary oedema may be due to decompensation of previously stable left-ventricular failure (eg with intercurrent illness), myocardial ischaemia/infarction, tamponade, arrhythmias, or hypertensive crisis (eg renal artery stenosis).

ABCDE approach

Signs and symptoms of cause

> History of hypertension, chest pain, collapse, palpitations
> Irregular pulse
> JVP elevated and rises on inspiration (tamponade)
> Blood pressure low (cardiac cause) or high (extracardiac)

Signs of severity

> Unable to talk in sentences/a few words
> Sat bolt upright
> White/pink frothy sputum
> Wheeze ('cardiac asthma')
> Crepitations throughout the chest

Immediate investigations as part of ABCDE

> Bloods, ABG, ECG, chest radiograph – **do not delay treatment**

Specific investigations

> Consider superurgent bedside echo if tamponade suspected

Immediate management as part of ABCDE

> Sit the patient up

Administer oxygen to keep SaO$_2$ 94–98% (start at 100%)

Specific management

> Opiates, eg diamorphine, as a venodilator and anxiolytic
> Intravenous furosemide, as a venodilator and diuretic
> Intravenous GTN as a venodilator and coronary vasodilator
> Intravenous digoxin if fast AF, as an inotrope and rate control
> Inhaled β agonists to reduce bronchospasm
> Consider need for non-invasive ventilation/intubation

Venodilators increase capacitance of the venous system and so reduce venous return and preload. Definitive therapy with diuretics, coronary reperfusion, antiarrhythmics, etc depends on the cause.

CASE 147

ACUTE SEVERE ASTHMA

Acute asthma can be life-threatening and come on with minimal provocation and little warning. Beware the asthmatic with a normal respiratory rate/$PaCO_2$ – are they improving or tiring?

ABCDE approach

Signs of severe exacerbation – any one of:

> PEFR 33–50% of best or predicted
> Tachypnoea >30 breaths/min
> Tachycardia >110 beats/min
> Unable to talk in complete sentences

Signs of life-threatening exacerbation – any one of:

> PEFR <33% of best or predicted
> Poor respiratory effort, exhaustion
> Arrhythmia
> Decreased conscious level
> Cyanosis
> Silent chest
> SaO_2 <92% or PaO_2 <8.0k Pa
> Normal/high $PaCO_2$ (should be **low** in hyperventilation)

Immediate investigations as part of ABCDE

> Bloods, ABG, ECG, chest radiograph – **do not delay treatment**

Immediate management as part of ABCDE

> Administer oxygen to keep SaO_2 94–98% (start at 100%)

Specific management

> Nebulised β agonists (drive nebuliser with oxygen)
> Consider back-to-back (continuous) nebulisers
> Nebulised ipratropium bromide (driven with oxygen)
> Steroids – prednisolone 40 mg or intravenous hydrocortisone
> Intravenous magnesium sulphate (if life-threatening)
> Early ICU referral if not improving/high $PaCO_2$

HYPERKALAEMIA

Patients with life-threatening hyperkalaemia may not look unwell, or have a clinically apparent cause of acute kidney injury, including renal failure as part of another acute illness, eg sepsis.

ABCDE approach

Signs of renal failure

> Tachypnoea (compensation for metabolic acidosis)
> Blood pressure low (prerenal) or high (glomerulonephritis)
> Low urine output/anuria

Signs of severity

> Tachycardia/arrhythmias

Immediate investigations as part of ABCDE

> Bloods, ABG, ECG, chest radiograph – **do not delay treatment**

Specific investigations

> Continuous ECG monitoring
> Urine dipstick
> Consider urinary catheter to monitor/treat obstruction

Immediate management as part of ABCDE

> Fluid resuscitation with non-K⁺-containing fluid if low BP
> Good intravenous access is vital – calcium is toxic if it extravasates

Specific management

Cardioprotection (takes 3–5 min, lasts 20 min to 1 h)

10 ml of 10% calcium chloride/gluconate if ECG shows changes of hyperkalaemia – changes should reverse within 5 min; if not, repeat

Shift K$^+$ into cells (takes up to 30 min, lasts 1–2 h)

Nebulised β agonists at high doses (10–20 mg)

50 ml of 50% dextrose with 10 units insulin over 20 min

Consider intravenous sodium bicarbonate if acidotic – aids insulin action and encourages kaliuresis

Remove K$^+$ from the body (takes hours, definitive)

Calcium resonium orally (with laxatives)/rectally

Furosemide for kaliuresis if passing urine (? + fluid)

Dialysis if unmanageable despite the above

Stop any K$^+$-raising drugs (ACE inhibitors, etc)

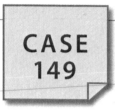

CASE 149 ANAPHYLAXIS

Anaphylaxis is a severe hypersensitivity reaction with rapidly developing airway and/or breathing and/or circulation problems.

ABCDE approach

Signs of anaphylaxis
History of exposure to a known anaphylatoxin
Flushing, urticaria, angioedema

Signs of severity
Airway swelling, stridor, hoarse voice
Cyanosis, respiratory exhaustion
Shortness of breath, wheeze
Tachycardia
Hypotension, sweaty/clammy
Acute confusion/decreased consciousness

Immediate investigations as part of ABCDE
Bloods, ABG, ECG, chest radiograph – **do not delay treatment**

Specific investigations to confirm anaphylaxis
Mast cell tryptase as soon as treatment under way, at 1–2 hours after onset of symptoms and at 24 hours after onset

Immediate management as part of ABCDE
Sit patients with airway/breathing problems upright
Lie patients with shock/circulatory collapse down
Administer oxygen to keep SaO_2 94–98% (start at 100%)
Fluid resuscitation – intravenous fluid challenge with 50–1000 ml

Specific management

Stop any suspected precipitant, eg new infusions

Do not induce vomiting after ingesting a precipitant

Intramuscular adrenaline 500 µg (0.5 mL of 1:1000)

Repeat after 5 min if no improvement

Intramuscular/intravenous chlorphenamine 10 mg

Intramuscular/intravenous hydrocortisone 200 mg

Consider inhaled/nebulised bronchodilators

Consider glucagon if suspected reaction to a β-blocker

Consider atropine if the patient becomes bradycardic

VIVA QUESTIONS

How would you break the news to someone that he or she had motor neurone disease?

Very importantly this should take place in a quiet environment, undisturbed and should be imparted by the most senior member of the medical team available, preferably with the nurse looking after the patient and an MND nurse specialist also present. It is probably best to give the patient advance notice that you are going to talk about the results of the investigations and encourage the patient to invite a family member to be there.

Most patients will probably not be familiar with motor neurone disease. It should be explained that it is a progressive condition affecting the nerves that supply the muscles, leading to wasting and weakness. They should be told that treatments are available that may slow the rate of progression of the disease, but that it cannot be cured. Explain that the cause remains unknown and that in the vast majority of cases it is not inherited/passed on to children.

Offer the patient and family literature/patient leaflets/websites about the condition, but do not foist these upon them. It is important to arrange a follow-up appointment in the near future, because undoubtedly they will have a lot of questions when they have had time to reflect upon the diagnosis and its implications.

What advice would you give to a patient going on a long-haul flight to Australia?

Assuming the patient is otherwise well they can be reassured that the risk of developing a DVT is low and can be minimised by taking the following steps:

> Regular movement of the feet/legs while sitting
>
> Taking frequent walks around the cabin
>
> Liberal consumption of non-alcoholic beverages
>
> Wearing well-fitting compression stockings
>
> The routine use of aspirin is not recommended (risk of bleed)

High-risk patients may need low molecular weight heparin prophylaxis – specialist advice should be sought.

Give me some causes of a raised/lowered sodium

Hypernatraemia is most commonly due to net water loss:

> Dehydration/inadequate fluid replacement/diarrhoea/diuretic use/insensible losses with fever/osmotic diuresis

Hyponatraemia is best considered in terms of the patient's extracellular fluid volume:

Hypovolaemic	Burns/diarrhoea/vomiting/pancreatitis/addisonism/cerebral or renal salt wasting
Euvolaemic	Sickle cell disease/hyperglycaemia/SIADH/ACTH deficiency/spurious (high serum protein/triglycerides)
Hypervolaemic	Cardiac failure/liver failure/renal (oedematous) failure/nephrotic syndrome

What do you understand by the term autosomal recessive?

Autosomal recessive disorders occur in patients whose healthy parents both carry the same recessive gene. The risk of recurrence for future pregnancies is 25% (1 in 4). Unlike autosomal dominant disorders there may be no family history of the disease.

Consanguinuity increases the risk of a recessive disorder because both parents are more likely to carry the same defective gene, carried by a common ancestor. Many of the inborn errors of metabolism are autosomal dominant disorders.

Tell me about the genetics of cystic fibrosis

Cystic fibrosis is the most common autosomal recessive disorder in northern Europeans; 1 in 20 of the population is a carrier, giving a disease frequency of approximately 1 in 2000 live births. Hundreds of different mutations in the cystic fibrosis gene on chromosome 7 have been found, but one common mutation (ΔF508) accounts for over 70% of cases.

When both parents are carriers there is a one in four risk of each pregnancy resulting in a child with cystic fibrosis. Precise prenatal diagnosis is possible and selective termination of affected pregnancies can be offered, if desired.

Discuss screening

Screening usually involves testing a large number of apparently healthy people to find those who have a specified disease or condition and those who do not. The sensitivity and specificity of the test will determine the success. It is usually thought to be ethical to screen only if there is an appropriate treatment available (eg cervical smears, mammography, Guthrie test).

What is the placebo response? How would you use it in a clinical trial?

The placebo is a positive therapeutic response by a patient when treated by an inactive, ineffective or sham therapy (physical, medical, psychological or surgical).

The clinical response to a placebo is compared with the response to the active treatment under study, usually with the patient and clinician ignorant as to which preparation the patient is taking (double blind). Only if there is a statistically significant benefit of the active treatment over placebo will the treatment be declared beneficial.

What is meant by a normal population?

This assumes for a given measurement that the population is distributed in a gaussian distribution (ie symmetrically in a bell-shaped curve with 95% within 2 standard deviations of the mean).

What do P values and confidence intervals represent?

P values represent the probability that a finding has occurred by chance, ie a P value of <0.05 (usually taken as statistically significant) means that there is a <5% chance that the result occurred by chance and >95% that it is real. Confidence intervals give a range in which the experimental result is likely to be in the general population (eg 95% chance that it will lie within the given range).

INDEX